Disclaimer

The information on this book is not intended to diagnose or treat any disease or condition. The authors are not a health practitioners and are not offering advice. No content in this book has been evaluated or approved by the FDA. Following any information is at your own risk.

Do your own thorough research before following any herbal advice. Be aware of interactions (drug or herbal), allergy, sensitivity or underlying conditions before proceeding with following any health information.

By continuing to read this book you agree to be responsible for yourself, do your own research, make your own choices and not to hold the authors responsible for your own actions.

Some of the plants, mentioned in the book, might be under protection in your area. Inform yourself and follow regional and national regulations, before you collect them.

Contents

3

Jolanta's Introduction

Why do I like this book?

Because it is so practical! You read about a herb and you know what to do with it. You suffer from.... a cold.... and you can help yourself with natural remedies. This is what I like in this book! Parish priest Johann Kuenzle wrote his book "Herbs and weeds" at the beginning of the 20th century for his parish people - ordinary people living in rural areas in the Swiss Alps. Life was different in those days, doctors and pharmacists were not around the corner and it was not unusual that parish priests and monks cared not only for the spirit and the soul, but also provided knowledge and medical help to those who needed it.

Father Künzle did more. In form of this booklet he provided knowledge so that people could help themselves.

He believed that there is everything people need on God's/ Nature's table. It is free, it is at hand, it is available to everybody, no matter how rich or poor, no matter whether educated or not. And, with this book, easy to read, written in the language of the locals, he encouraged people to use wild herbs: those which could heal and those, delicious ones which could be added to food so that people stay healthier and happier.

The booklet was like a snowball rolling down the slope of a mountain and turning into a huge avalanche. The first one appeared in 1911. It was so popular that one edition followed another topping up to over two million copies sold. In those days! In a small country like Switzerland! When, during the Spanish flu, not a single person died in the Priest's parish, his popularity grew even faster. Johann Künzle adapted his booklet for children, and it was included into the curriculum of the local schools. Later in his life he wrote many books on herbs, including "The great herbal book" where he described over 100 herbs and the ways how to use them.

But here we have this small booklet.

Why do I like this book?

Because it is for those who love nature, who live with nature and from nature. It is for me! And for you! It is almost a hundred years old. That is true, but herbs do not become outdated in a hundred years. They are neither a computer, nor a car. They have existed for may be even longer than we humans and they will continue growing and thriving if we, humans, leave their habitats untouched. When I was reading and translating the book, I was so happy to discover that I can still find all the plants mentioned in the book in my garden, in the meadow nearby, in the forest just 200 meters away and up in the Alps.

This booklet transports the reader into the beginning of the 20th Century. One can feel the atmosphere, sense how people lived, how they worked, how they treated children, what was important in those days. He loved ordinary people. They were his heroes, his examples of good practice: the food they ate, the herbs they used, the way they dressed and hardened their bodies.
And then there were the other ones, already influenced by the vanity of this world... here the voice of Father Künzle was stricter. If you follow fashions in eating, those nicely packed unhealthy foods or loads of meat served on nice different plates and disregard health - you would be told off. Even the chocolate got his portion of criticism.

Father Kuenzle believed in the strength and power of plants growing in the wild nature under harsh conditions. The best herbs, he said, are the ones that grow high up and are hard to reach. If you reach them, you have the best! One can understand it also figuratively. You do not get the best quality if you do not put any effort. You do not have good health if you do not put in effort: grow or collect your own herbs/food, be physically active in healthy surroundings, harden your body and soul, develop a spiritual life.

When Johann Künzle refers to ailments and illnesses, I find his approach very up to date and modern, because the first question is - what was the reason for the pain, the inflammation, the stiffness. "What does the body lack?"

And then it was followed by the next question: "What help does the body need?" He was not going to give advice or remedies for symptoms before knowing the reason. If it is a headache or poor digestion - what is the reason for it? Unhealthy meal, too little physical activity, too weak immune system... only then the advice will follow.

There is a saying that something new is the forgotten old. Nowadays we hear more and more of body cleansing therapies. Father Künzle was promoting that a hundred years ago. We hear more and more about the usefulness of fasting - this is what he strongly promotes in this book.

People keeping animals, farmers raising cattle might find quite a few useful pieces of advice here as well.

Of course, nowadays the conditions are different. One would not even think of treating serious illnesses like tuberculosis without modern medicine. Of course, you go to your doctor, of course you ask for his or her advice, but would we not be much more resistant to viruses, bacteria, various ailments like sore throats or cough, or constipation if we introduced more herbs into our lives? This is how I personally use the advice in this book - I use herbs to stay healthy.

The qualities of these wild growing herbs have not changed in 100 years. We, humans, have changed, we have forgotten what our forefathers knew, we got carried away by readymade food or factory-made medicine, but the memory of what is genuine and real is still there and it is never too late to turn back and catch up with what we used to know.

Actually, food and medicine is one and the same. This is how I see it. And this is nothing new. Many remember the famous quote by Greek physician Hippocrates, "Let food be thy medicine, and let medicine be thy food". When I use Herbs for food, I do not need medicine. We are part of nature, whether we like it or not. Our bodies are composed of the same substances, like trees, flowers, herbs. When I give enough natural and varied food to my body, my body knows better than I do what I need for my brain, muscles, good eyesight, healthy skin, healthy sleep... and take a bit of potassium from this plant, a bit of magnesium from that one, Vitamin C or A, or B from the third... The body knows what it needs and what it does not need comes out in a natural way and regularly. How many different natural plants do we get in supermarkets? Let's take salad. How many different herbs for salad do we get? 2? May be 5? And how many herbs suitable for salad are there in nature? 10? 25? 100? Those in supermarkets are grown as monoculture protected by herbicides, pesticides, fungicides. Those in nature have to protect themselves against all creepy crawlers, against fungus, bacteria and viruses and the survivors have all the strength and the power which we get by consuming them as food. If we add them to our salad, we get all the protective ingredients they contain.

Of course, one has to know what one puts in one's mouth. One has to be confident and pick only the herbs one knows. And this is what this book is about! It tells us about medical and culinary herbs.

I myself am a herbalist. I am teaching herbs, I am growing, collecting, using herbs as food and medicine, experimenting, sharing the knowledge and I am using Father Künzle's book as a practical teaching material.

The herbal knowledge came not only from books and courses. I still remember my grandmother collecting St John's wort and hanging it in the attic to dry. She introduced many herbs to me. Now it is my turn to pass on the knowledge.

When I talk to women and men in my herbal workshops, they do know, they do recognize many herbs, they do use some of them, they bring back the old names for this or that herb, they just need encouragement to use herbs again.

I am not against doctors and modern medicine. We need it. We need the research and understanding why, we need diagnosis - this is what modern medicine is very good at, we need help when accidents happen, epidemics break out, when children are born.... but I do not believe in excess of food supplements when nature is around, I do not believe in swallowing antibiotics for a simple cold or painkillers without finding a reason for the pain. I believe that we are responsible for our health. My health is MY health.

It is important to find out the reason and then it is in our hands to decide what to do with the diagnosis. In this age of information one can choose different ways: changing one's way of life? Changing what one eats? Introducing more physical activities? Spending more time in nature?

In this world of information, we have to find our own way, especially when it concerns us personally, our lives, lives of our children, our health. We have to take information with a critical mind. The same applies to this book. This is one way of seeing and using herbs. I compare what I read in this book with what I know from other books. E.g. I have learned not to boil herbs, as boiling kills a lot of useful substances. Father Kuenzle advises to boil the herbs. Well, through boiling one loses some substances, but gets more of other substances. One needs to find out more. I have learned that by making tinctures and herbal oils one should keep jars away from the sun. Father Kuenzle suggests keeping them in the sun. When I started asking local people, I found many who would develop e.g. Arnica tincture or St John's oil in the sun. I love experimenting. I will try out and compare.

Much research has been done on herbs lately. In many cases research confirms what has been known for ages, in some cases it finds some "dangerous substances" in a herb and, all of a sudden, the herb is downgraded. But the dosage makes a difference between medicine and poison whether one uses herbs or whether one uses tablets. It is important to learn, find out, read, study, and make one's own decisions based on knowledge.

I hope you will find the book as useful and interesting to read as I did and that it might, somehow contribute to positive changes in your lives or give you a glimpse into the world 100 years ago. And, if you develop a wish to see all the herbs mentioned in the book, book a holiday in the Swiss or Austrian Alps. The herbs are still here! There are still spots of untouched nature.

And, if you need a guide, I will happily help you discover these treasures on the God's laid table.

Judson's Foreword

I first became aware of Fr. Künzle through the works of Maria Treben. Mrs. Treben was an Austrian herbalist who became quite famous in the 1970s. She wrote several excellent books and was a popular public speaker. In large part, she gave back to the western world the tradition of German Folk Medicine. After the fall of the Roman Empire, the knowledge of civilization, the history, the religious texts... the books and yes, the herbs and their medicinal use, was preserved by certain monks and priest, especially in Central Europe and Ireland. It has often been said, that "the Irish saved civilization" in this manner, but it is equally true of the Germanic and Slavic peoples. Such is especially the case with Herbal Medicine.

Among the first herbals written in the post Greek and Roman eras was by an monk named Walafrid Strabo. Abbot Strabo was born around 800 AD. He grew to be among the most respected and learned men of his era. He was influential in what one may call "Church Politics", a theologian and tutor to the offspring of Emperor Charlemagne. He spent his later years in an idyllic setting, a monastery in Germany, where he wrote a charming book called, Hortulus. Hortulus was a book of poetry describing the medicinal herbs and their uses that he grew in his little garden. It is full of wit and good humor, and really stands on its own as a masterpiece of the era. This was a time when monasteries and nunneries were mandated, by Papal decree, to have "physick gardens" and to operate charitable hospitals. Monks, nuns and priests were often educated and skilled in herbal medicine. Today, when we look at the Latin name of an herb and see the term "officinalis", that is still an indication that it was an herb officially used in the Middle Ages by the Monastic herbalist.

The tradition of Monastic Medicine reached its greatest height in the 1100s, when a German nun, Saint Hildegard von Bingen, began to write on herbal medicine. Although, she would have been steeped in the herbal tradition of her order, Saint Hildegard was a visionary. She received messages from angels, saints and, "The Voice of The Living Light." Her works include the largest body of religious music composed in the Middle Ages, most of which is still heard in Catholic Churches today. She wrote books on theology that are so remarkably profound as to qualify her a Doctor of the Church. She wrote two books on herbal medicine and horticulture that are both spiritual and practical. She seemed to have the Wisdom of Solomon, and like Solomon, people came from all over Europe to learn from her. This frail, middle aged woman, so sickly and beset by illness that she had been often blind and bed-ridden as a youth, and unable to receive a formal education, became recognized as the wisest person on earth during the second half of her life. She was in great demand as a speaker, and as her body seemed to strengthen and heal along with the mission she was given to impart the knowledge she received, she was asked by the Pope and Bishops to preach and teach in as many Catholic Churches in Central Europe as she could reach.

With the ebbs and flows of history and political upheaval for which Central Europe is so rightly known, much was not written down over the centuries, and the Monastic Medicine became "folk medicine." This deep and rich herbalism became part of the lives of common people. The term, "kitchen medicine" came into use for the teas and poultices one would employ to treat ailments within the family.

In the 1800s, a new force came on the scene. The dynamic and brilliant Father Sebastian Kneipp became, arguably, the most famous herbalist in the western world! While a seminary student, the future Fr. Kneipp contracted tuberculosis. His case was dire, and no medical treatment could help. He was informed by doctors, in no uncertain terms, that he would die before he graduated. Although, Fr. Kneipp was likely well steeped in the German Folk Medicine tradition even as a youth, it was advice he found in an old book that proved to be his cure. The book advised the sick to "toughen the constitution" by swimming regularly in cold water. The young Fr. Kneipp did so, daily swimming in the frigid river... and his condition improved. A fellow seminarian was even sicker than he, so he began bringing his friend along on his daily swims. Soon, both young men were fully recovered, healthy and ready for graduation! This led to Fr. Kneipp's classic book, My Water Cure.

My Water Cure was a book of instruction on the systematic use of (mostly) cold water baths that Fr. Kneipp developed in treating the multifarious illnesses of his parishioners. It was also, a comprehensive herbal. Fr. Kneipp's stated goal was to provide an apothecary, and instructions for use, for the common man. His vision was the ideal of German Folk Medicine: Children, having been thoroughly instructed by their parents, gathering herbs from among the wildflowers, as they walked barefoot in the morning dew. Kitchens, fully stocked with well ordered and properly prepared herbs. Parents, acting as effective physicians for their families, and passing on that wisdom.

My Water Cure Became the first international "best seller". The book was so popular that flawed counterfeits were sold in multiple languages. Even today, as Jolanta can attest, Fr. Kneipp's cold water therapies are still popular among people in her region, and his more elaborate treatments are performed in spas that are a regular part of life in her beautiful part of the world.

Many were inspired by Fr. Kneipp. Chief among them was Fr. Künzle. It is likely that Fr. Künzle's small book on "herbs and weeds" would have even outsold Fr. Kneipp's book of a generation earlier, had it been translated into English, French, Spanish, etc, and have been able to reach beyond the region in which it was published. But, then came the wars.... back to back, "world wars". Was it likely that with anti-German sentiment so high in America, France and England, that an herbal written in the German language, even by a Swiss priest, would be popular? No, especially in mostly protestant America and England.... and, especially not as herbal medicine was being outlawed in much of the "modern world."

The 1920s brought into enforcement the Pure Foods and Drugs Act to America, outlawing "snake oil", and all treatments not approved by the modern medical community... the allopathic medical practitioners, the scientists who only believe what can be seen under a microscope and proven in a laboratory. Never mind if an herb has been successfully used to treat an illness for over 2,000 years.... it must now be rejected in favor of a pill from a pharmaceutical company. Fr. Künzle fought such bureaucracies in his time and won a landmark victory when he showed that he could treat diabetes more effectively than the doctors of his day. If only we had a man of his renown, expertise and fighting spirit today, when out rights to use traditional, herbal medicine are being restricted more than ever!

"Snake Oil", by the way, was based on the herb, Echinacea.... which is still a better treatment for the tissue damage caused by venomous snakes and certain spiders than anything the drug companies have been able to invent! Would that we could bring back the old fashioned "Medicine Shows" where "patent", generally herbal based, medicines were sold by flamboyant barkers, in between the organic musical performances that birthed both country music and jazz! Throw in a few clowns and jugglers, and that sure beats going to the doctor! "Buyer beware" is sage advice…. otherwise, we are doomed to ignorance, fewer options and ever higher prices.

When I first encountered Mrs. Treben's books, Health from God's Garden and Heath Through God's Pharmacy, they seemed very familiar. The Appalachian Mountains of North Carolina, where I was born, are historically Scots-Irish and Cherokee. But, those mountains were also a haven for many Germans, Swiss, Polish, Alpine Italian, etc. folks, who either fled the World Was as refuges, or immigrated here for other reasons… such as the skiing that was popular in the 1960s/70s. The "Alpine" style was very much in fashion in architecture and decoration as I grew up, and such accents were common. My family knew many such immigrants as the one who saved a small child's life when she stumbled into a hornet's nest, sucking out the venom before an ambulance could arrive. Or, the old park ranger I met when I was a teen… a first generation German-American, raised on Kneipp practices and German Folk Medicine, who had experienced only one cold in his nearly 80 years, and could hike rugged terrain at a faster pace than me, talking the entire time! My own herbal training was very much in the Scots-Irish, British and Native American traditions… and, although I spent a decade or so studying Traditional Chinese Medicine, German Folk Medicine was always at hand.

Mrs. Treben's books became favorites and I recommend them to both beginners and to experienced herbalists. I began researching the authors she mentioned. That led me to Saint Hildegard and Fr. Kneipp. One name kept coming up though, and that was that of Fr. Künzle. Thanks to the internet, I was able to find out who he was. But, no English translation of his works either existed or was still in print. I don't know why, exactly, that I became drawn to German Folk Medicine... perhaps it is the precision and ease with which the Germanic writers describe herbs and explain their uses. Perhaps, it is the reverence and joy with which they practice their craft. Perhaps, it is just because the world outside their doors is so very similar to mine.

Jolanta and I met on The Grow Network Forums. I quickly recognized her as a skilled and experienced herbalist, in the tradition to which I was being drawn. So, I asked her if she would be interesting in collaborating on this book. To my surprise, she did... and, we have spent days and months enjoying and discussing this great work. All credit for the translation goes to Jolanta. I handled the publishing and offered my perspective when I think it may be helpful for American readers. The photos are courtesy of Jolanta and her husband.

We are pleased to revive this work that is far too important to be forgotten. We hope that Fr. Künzle would be pleased. We hope that our readers will also explore Fr. Kneipp's works, as we are both practitioners of the Kneipp tradition. Saint Hildegard von Bingen, pray for us. And, of course, this Irish-American Catholic must also invoke Saint Fiachre! Above all though, we hope you will find something of use in this work. We both live in the mountains, although nearly half a world apart. The same plants mostly grow in both of our regions. We find health in peaceful walks and living with the seasons, using the herbs and food God provided in our lands... which, if they be somewhat more harsh than the Garden of Eden, can be no less beautiful. We wish you good health... and a serving of sauerkraut!

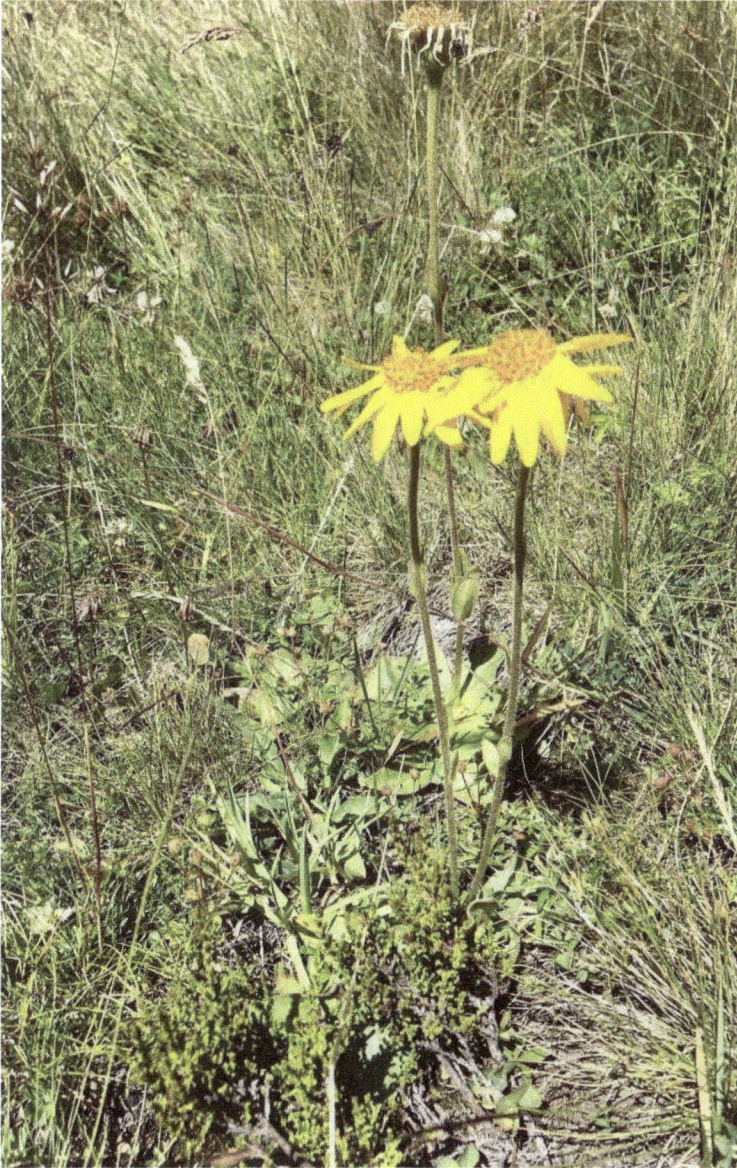

Arnica

Arnica (arnica montana)

is recommended by all herbalists, especially by Pastor Kneipp himself for wounds, it prevents suppuration and bleeding and accelerates healing.

It also works wonderfully on sprains, dislocations and swellings that result from them.

Preparation: Arnica flowers are put in alcohol, exposed to the sun or otherwise to the warmth for 10 days, then strained, and the tincture is ready.

In the case of open wounds, this tincture must be diluted with water so that you take three tablespoons per liter of water. It can be used unmixed for sprains.

JW: In my neighborhood here in the Austrian Alps one can find Arnica tincture or oil in many houses. In the mountain area where almost everybody goes skiing, hiking, mountain biking, strains, bumps, etc. happen relatively often. The home remedy - Arnica tincture is of great help in many cases.

I love Arnica. It is a beautiful mountain flower. The odor is so gentle. Unfortunately, its habitat is getting smaller with every new ski lift. In Tirol where I live, it is a already a protected plant.

I use Arnika tincture and Arnica oil. For external use only. Tincture applied for a longer time may dry out the skin. This is when oil helps. Arnica oil is made in the same way as Johann Künzle recommended to make Arnica tincture. One uses high quality oil instead of alcohol. There are differences in how long one should keep tincture or oil in the sun. Some recipes say only 8 days, some, up to 6 weeks. Some keep tincture and oil in the sun, some protect it from the sun. Well, as long as everybody is satisfied with home made oil and tincture, all ways are good. By

the way, Arnica oil is also a good basis for making ointments or salves.

Before you start experimenting with Arnica, find out whether you are not allergic to plants from the Asteraceae family.

JC: Although Arnica should generally not be used internally, under proper guidance from a qualified herbalist, it may be useful for internal use in certain heart conditions such as angina and heart failure, and to strengthen the immune system. Used externally, Arnica reduces inflammation and helps stop bleeding, while increasing local blood supply. As a homeopathic remedy, Arnica is quite effective against internal bleeding, all manner of injuries and shock.

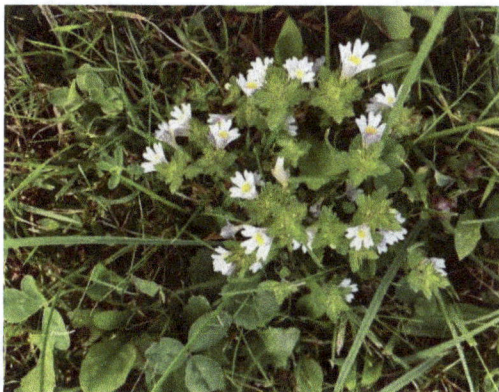

Eyebright

Eyebright (Euphrasia)

was known as an excellent means of strengthening the eyes even before the birth of Christ. The ancients boiled it with wine and drank it regularly before going to bed. Fr. Kneipp recommends a decoction of eyebright, just washing your eyes diligently with eyebright water decoction. This herb is by far most effective when you throw it into a jar or in the barrel where you are fermenting cider, let it ferment with the drink and drink it throughout the year.

Fr. Kneipp also recommends the herb for the stomach.

JW: Eyebright is so tiny that you really have to know what you are looking for to find it. But, when you take it into your hand, you feel that the plant is strongly built. It has a strong stem and robust leaves. Eyebright is well adapted to live under harsh conditions. It knows that, being so small, it cannot get all the necessary substances itself, that is why its roots are fixed to the roots of other plants. It is a semi parasitic plant. But not a danger to the host plants. They all thrive together. So far, I have only admired it in nature - used for the pleasure of eyes, rather than for the sight, but I know people who use Eyebright infusions for eye baths.

JC: Here, we have the first mention of Father Sebastian Kneipp, a great hero of mine and one of my favorite herbalists. I think it necessary to mention that both Frs. Kneipp and Künzle were great herbal healers and as essential to the folk medicine tradition of the German speaking world as Saint Hildegard von Bingen or Abbot Walafrid Strabo... as essential as Hippocrates and Dioscorides to the Greek tradition. As for Eyebright, the small and beautiful flower, it does reduce inflammation and mucus in the eyes. It also reduces mucus in the sinuses and lungs. The herb is astringent but also aids in digestion.

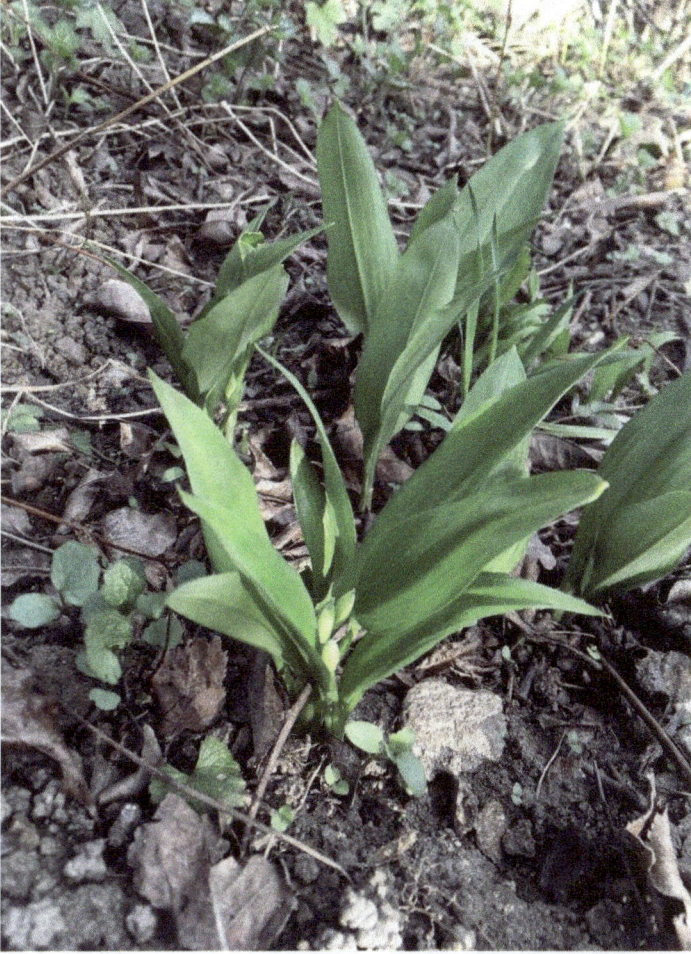

Ramsons

Ramsons, Wild garlic (Allium ursinum),

 In our god-blessed mountains, wild and in abundance grows a wonderful, blood-cleansing herb, the wild garlic, called Ramsons or as it is called in this part of the world: Rämschelen or Rimschelen. It tastes like strong chives, looks like the leaves of the dog rose, but is immediately recognized by its taste. In March it starts appearing in rich soil in shady places, under trees, under hedges and at the edges of forests, etc., from down in the valley up to the Alps. You cut the wild garlic like chives and throw a lot of it into the soup; many eat it and prepare it just like salad. It cleans the whole body, drives out sick, tangled substances, makes the blood healthy, drives away and kills toxic substances.

The herb dies in June and disappears.

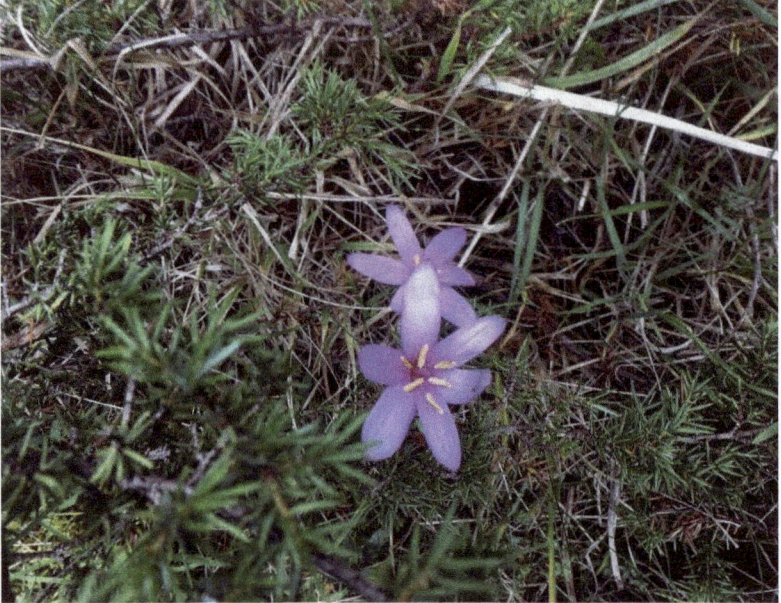

Meadow Saffron

Children and unexperienced are never to be sent out to collect Ramsons, as they could easily bring home the poisonous and deadly meadow saffron (Colchicum). The taste of the Ramson is the safest identification for the unexperienced people, as this plant smells like garlic, which is not the case with the Meadow Saffron.

Permanently sick people, people with eczema and abscesses,

pale people and rheumatics should worship wild garlic like gold, as well as chives, garlic and onions. The Jews certainly owe the tenacity and perseverance of their race partly thanks to their 4,000-year-old habit of eating garlic. The well-known and famous Alpine leek (Allium victorialis) is also a leek variety and therefore has its power.

JW: I like garlic and I like ramsons. Unfortunately, Ramsons do not like the conifer forests surrounding our village. They prefer deciduous trees or mixed woods. I have to travel to the beech forests in Bavaria to collect them and it needs good timing, as you can find and collect them only for a short time in spring. Then they disappear, as these spring herbs later would not get any sun under thick beech foliage. They use the time slot in spring before the trees develop their leaves.

Father Künzle warned that there is a danger of collecting some poisonous plants instead of ramsons. That is very true. One of the poisonous plants, looking very much like ramsons is the Lily-of-the-Valley (convallaria majalis). It also grows in spring. It also likes deciduous forests. Father Künzle writes that you recognize the right ones by the garlic taste. That is true, but once you have a few ramsons in your hands everything smells garlic, including the wrongly picked herbs, so be careful. Collect ramsons only if you are absolutely sure that you are taking the right ones.

JC: In the Appalachian Mountains of the American southeast where I live, Ramsons are called "ramps". Our ramps are very short lived, and only harvested around Easter. They are my favorite wild plant food. I actually salivate at the thought of them. The ramps are sweet and mildly warming. Eaten raw, they cause one to smell strongly of garlic, leeks or onions with just the slightest perspiration. This strong scent is evidence of the powerful medicinal action of these delicious alliums! The old folks say they are a spring tonic, blood cleanser and immune booster. Frankly, even if they were bad for you…. I'd eat as many as I could get! You can use them as you would green onions/scallions. An excellent condiment can be made like a pesto – finely chop your ramps (leave the bulb and use the leaves if possible, so they will re-grow), add salt, olive oil and dried crushed red pepper. I find this the ideal complement to an Easter ham, especially with blue cheese!

Pimpinella

What is Pimpinella? It is known to many people under the name "Goat root" as it spreads like billy goats. It blooms like caraway and chervil and can be found in abundance from May onwards from down in the valley up to the high Alps; one uses the roots which are finely chopped up, dried and powdered in a coffee grinder. The powder can then be enjoyed in coffee, milk, wine, cider or water.

Pimpinella is as violent as a Russian and chases away tangled and thick substances and festering substances from the larynx, lungs, stomach, intestines, cures hoarseness (boiled in wine, gargled and drunk) in one hour, therefore invaluable for speakers, removes intestinal and pulmonary catarrh.

When the Indians in Dakota want to be very friendly to someone, they give them a handful of this Pimpinella which is very rare in their area.

We have produced Pimpinella candies from Pimpinella powder. It is very useful for hoarseness, coughs, catarrh, pulmonary and stomach congestion.

JC: Pimpinella is diaphoretic, which means it helps break a fever. It is also a diuretic, meaning it helps reduce bodily fluids through increasing urine. It settles the stomach. It also reduces inflammation. The root has a hot quality that helps with toothache, sore throat and bronchitis.

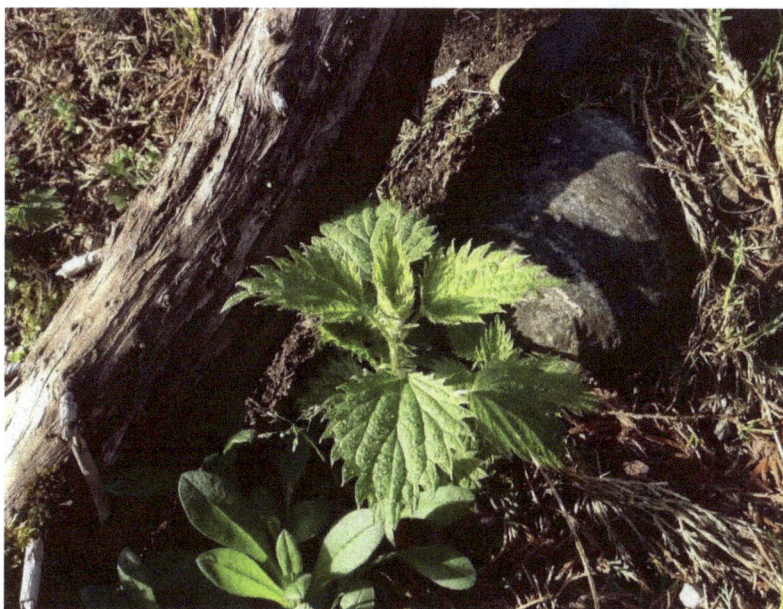
Stinging Nettle

The nettle (aurtica dioica and urens)

resembles a "ruchen cholderi" a man with grim looks but with a helpful heart who in an emergency would save the life of a neighbour by sacrificing his own.

  Why did God give this plant fire? First of all, so that people know them; I have met a lot of town people who do not know a single plant apart from the nettle, "it's really like that", but they are competent in lace, fringes, corsets and perfumeries. Secondly, so that it is not wiped out by the little animals, because everything from the young calf to the smallest snail would chew and eat it out because for them they taste like the finest chocolate. Fire is a prohibition sign that every goat can read.

Everything on this plant is used, from the roots to the seeds. The root, boiled in vinegar, is by far the best remedy for hair growth. The herb cleanses the lungs, stomach, intestines and has a healing effect when used for a longer time on gastric and intestinal ulcers. In this case you prepare it with plantain and juniper and thyme (well boiled) and drink it warm (a sip several times a day).

For livestock, nettle, along with juniper, is the number one medicine; animals like to eat it dry; it cleanses the stomach and intestines. When boiled green it is a means of keeping the pigs healthy.

The external application of the nettle is not very popular; however, I know people who, when rheumatism sets in, whip the painful areas with nettles and are free of pain.

The nettle should be approached like sensitive, irritable people and therefore they should be touched only with gloves.

JW: The nettle is one of my favorite herbs. I use it like many other herbs to detoxify and to strengthen my body. This is an excellent herb to show how food can be medicine and medicine can be food. In spring I cook nettle soup, in early summer I collect leaves for my detox herbal teas - I prefer to drink this tea in the morning as it is a diuretic; in late summer I collect nettle seeds - my super food giving energy, joy of life throughout the winter; and in autumn I collect roots for rinsing my hair. I use it in the same way as Father Künzle recommended - I boil it in homemade apple vinegar.

Do you know that there are male and female nettles? A group of male ones would grow not too far away from the female ones. But they do not mix. I collect seeds from the female plants, of course.

Every nettle stings, that is true, but there is a way of approaching it without gloves. If you stroke it from down upwards, you will not be stung. The nettle is prepared to fight enemies from above, not from under.

This is how I collect nettle seeds - this superfood which can be added to soup, porridge, any herbal drink, sprayed on bread and butter or baked in bread or buns... or (my favorite way) just taking half a teaspoon of it once a day.

I find female nettles, cut the top part with seeds, spread them on a sheet in a shade in a dry place, wait, until seeds start falling off, stroke the seeds (with latex gloves) off the stem and put them into jars.

I never throw away the rest. A nettle is an excellent fertilizer for garden plants. Actually, my only fertilizers are nettle, comfrey and horsetail.

JC: Aside from being a delicious food plant, Nettles have a great effect in the treatment of nasal allergies. Maria Treben recommended Nettle Tea with Swedish Bitters for that purpose, and I have found it an excellent remedy. Moreover, Nettles cleanse the blood, reduce the symptoms of arthritis, are high in iron and good for the treatment of anemia, are a tonic for the immune system, and good for everything from gout to eczema to hemorrhoids. If one were only to harvest one wild plant for health and nutrition, the Stinging Nettle would be a top contender... and easy to identify!

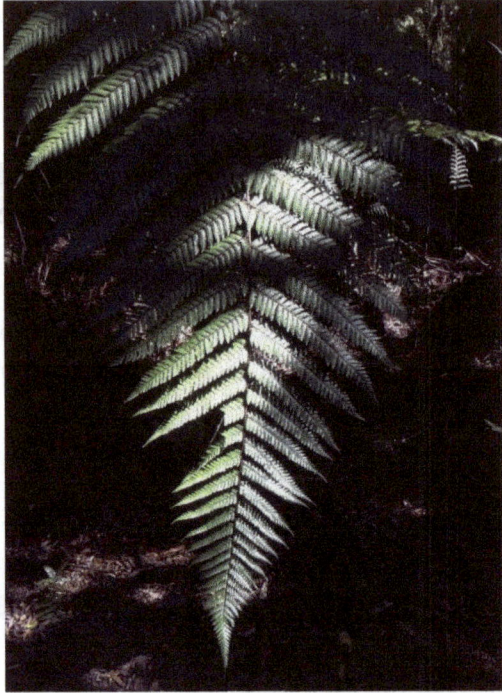

Fern

The fern (Aspidium filix)

What is the best bed for people suffering from cramps, aching limbs, rheumatism, rheumatic toothache, rheumatic headache? A sack filled with dried fern. Fern draws these things out and gives relief to those who suffer. In addition, fleas and bed bugs flee miles and miles away from such a bed, and nothing can induce them to return as long as a bag filled with fern is there.

Saddlers would make good business by stuffing mattresses with dried fern instead of seaweed.

All, even the smallest varieties of fern, used internally (but only in small doses and mixed with 3/4 wine) drive away worms.

The large fern root (weighs up to 2 kilos) has an astonishing, almost wonderful effect against all the ailments mentioned above. Foot baths in this root, used for 8 to 14 days, cure the most severe convulsive and gouty ailments. Full baths made from this root are even more effective. The large fern root, boiled in vinegar and rubbed in, drives away rheumatic stiffness etc.

Thus the despised fern, which is used like straw, is a great, glorious gift from God for suffering mankind.

Ferns in the shoes relieve tiredness and provide warm feet.

In case of rheumatism, lumbago, aching limbs, a sudden stiffness, one immediately fetches a right bundle of green fern leaves and puts it on the painful area; at the beginning the pain increases, but then it disappears.

When the hearing loss comes from cold and draft, and is therefore rheumatic, one should stuff the pillow with green fern leaves and sleep on it. It is even better to put fern seeds into a very small sack and stuff it into your ears. The seeds can be seen on the lower side of the fern leaves in rows of black spots and they fall off as fine black dust when ripe.

In the winter, a tincture of fern is used for rubbing it in; it is made by chopping green leaves, placing them in a glass, pouring alcohol over them until the fern is covered, sealing well and exposing it to the sun or to the warmth for 4-6 days; then the spirit which has now become fern tincture is poured off. Eucalyptus oil is just as good.

The best of the ferns is the Male fern (Aspidium filix), called Falegata by the Romans and Filice by the Italians. The farmers call it feather fern, ostrich fern. The leaves have no secondary branches and are like palm leaves; the Male fern thrives in moist forests in rich soil and is often grown in gardens.

The forest moss, especially the stagshorn moss (Lycopodium), which produces meter-long stems, has the same power against cramps and spasmodic legs as the fern root. The decoction can be used repeatedly for foot-baths. The stagshorn moss decoction drives away all kinds of lice and vermin from people and cattle.

A bundle of stagshorn moss at the foot of the bed, pulls cramps out of the legs, probably because this plant contains radium.

JC: There are many types of fern and some are more appropriate for internal use than others. For centuries, the Bracken Fern has been eaten as a spring delicacy, but now they say it could be slightly carcinogenic. Well, in all honestly... "they" say many herbs that have been in common use for centuries may cause cancer, such as comfrey and sassafras. When one really looks at those studies, one finds such high concentrations of the herb used in experiments on rats that the human would have a very difficult time replicating such results in real life. Popular herbalist, Dr. Patrick Jones, is fond of saying that what he learned from such studies is not to give massive amounts of comfrey to baby rats! That caveat given, we are legally encouraged to give such warnings. The Maidenhair Fern has been used traditionally in for coughs. The Hart's Tongue Fern was especially recommended by Saint Hildegard for the liver, lungs and painful intestines, but is now rare and protected in many nations. She recommended other ferns for everything from rheumatism to demonic possession. The Lady Fern is said to reduce labor pains during childbirth and increase the flow of milk afterward. At least 68 fern varieties are mentioned as useful either for herbal medicine or food in the books on my shelf. These useful plants warrant much more exploration by the modern herbalist.

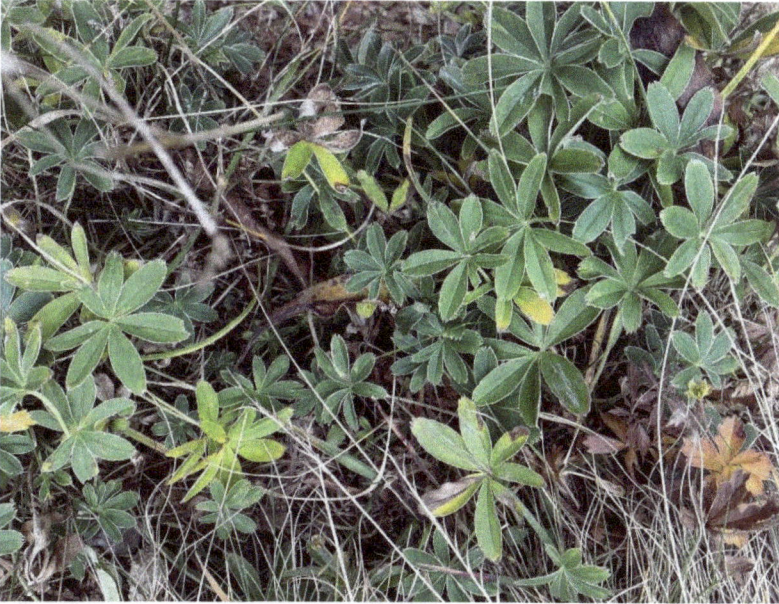

Alpine Lady's Mantle

The Lady's Mantle (Alchymilla vulgaris) or Dew's Mantle, Mantle herb, God Mother's Mantle, Help for Women, All women healer.

The name alone indicates already part of the healing power of this herb. It thrives everywhere on the shady side, on streams, somewhat damp meadows, especially on the mountains up to the snow line.

It has an elegant, noble sister: the alpine lady's-mantle (Alchymilla alpina), which has the same properties to an even greater extent;

However, this only thrives in the Alpine region and is recognizable by its silver sheen.

The ancients knew the healing power of this plant very well and gave it the name Alchymilla (magic herb).

The lady's mantle, well boiled and drunk warm, relieves headache, heals cold in the head, eye infections, and often headaches, toothaches (gargle your mouth!)

It also heals fever, burns, suppuration and ulcers, which is why it cannot be more than enough recommended to women. Every woman after giving birth should diligently drink quite a lot of this herb for 8 to 10 days. Some children would still have their mother and many a beaten widower his wife if they had known this gift of God.

Furthermore, the herb, boiled and drunk a lot, takes fever and burns in case of broken ribs, knocks from wood, stone, iron, after severe falls. A great many people die from internal injuries; this herb quickly removes fever and burn, and speeds healing; but in this case drink a lot, 1 to 2 liter a day, depending on thirst. (Add sugar!)

Externally applied and crushed, lady's mantle heals wounds, stabs, cuts.

Children who always have weak muscles despite eating well will become strong with continued use of this tea.

The lady's mantle, drunk as tea, cures the diarrhea. This herb is of the highest value for cattle; fed dry, it heals diarrhea.

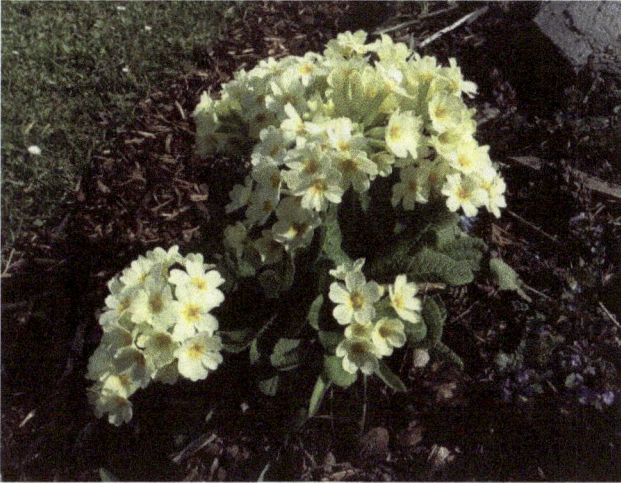

Cowslip

The tea from the lady's mantle is lovely and pleasant; mixed with cowslip (Primula Veris), it is even better than Chinese tea and is far healthier than this; it calms nerves and provides sound sleep and is a quick remedy for people who often get nauseous.

In case of obesity and a bloated body, provided this is not due to abundant food and lack of exercise, the alpine lady's-mantle (Alchymilla alpina) offers help if it is used for a long time. Collect lady's mantle from May to July, dry it well in the sun and keep it dry!

What a healing power has the benevolent Creator bestowed on this delicate herb.

JW: I am a woman, thus I always make sure that I have enough dried Lady's mantle at home to last throughout a year. When I go on mountain tours, I bring home the Alpine lady's mantle which we call a silver mantle. It really has a silver shine and is believed to be much more powerful than the green one.

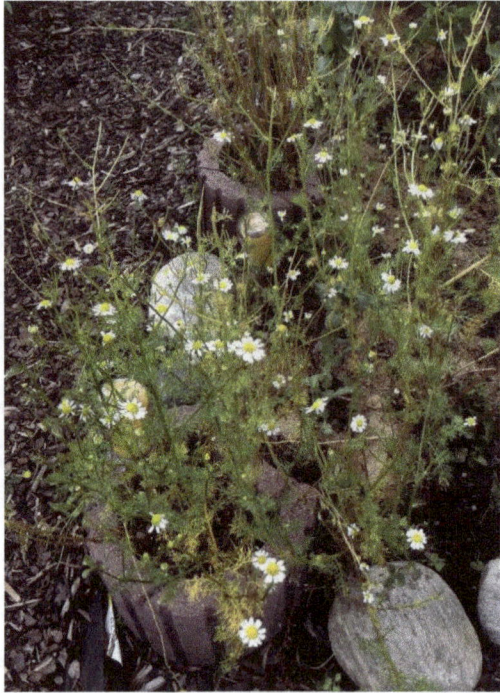

Chamomile

Women drink lady's Mantle tea after a child's birth; for menstruation cramps (in a mixture with chamomile and/or fennel, or caraway seeds). For menopause women prefer the Alpine one, often in a mixture with red clover (trifolium pratense).

Lady's mantle' taste is quite boring, that is why I would mix it with other "female" herbs like lemon balm, lavender or rose petals, or, as Father Künzle recommended with cowslip - this gently smelling spring herb which calms down the nerves, when needed.

Have you heard of and seen the magic water drop in the middle of the leave? No, it is not a drop of dew. It comes from the inside of the herb. There are many stories and legends about this drop. They say that Cleopatra washed her face with these drops... that alchemists used it as heaven water... I drink this drop when I see one.

JC: Lady's Mantle is listed as alterative, which means it restores proper function of the body, gradually bringing one back to health. It is antirheumatic, referring to the swelling of joints such as in arthritis. It is astringent (tightening or restoring tone to tissue) and diuretic (reducing fluid). It is an emmenagogue, meaning that it stimulates menstruation by increasing blood flow. The herb is febrifuge (breaks a fever), sedative (calming), styptic (helps stop bleeding), tonic (strengthening/balancing) and vulnerary (meaning it helps heal wounds). Few plants offer more benefit, especially to women.

Goldenrod (Solidago virga aurea)

You will find this perennial, often a meter-high plant, with yellow flowers in deforested places, berry places, along roadsides. It rightly deserves the name goldenrod.

Internally one uses the tea for croup, sore throat, bladder ailments, light diarrhea, sleeplessness, but for the internal use one should always add the same amount of juniper berries or common centaury; take half a cup three to five times a day.

The soaked dry herb is also used as poultices for the same diseases externally.

The two alpine relatives senecio cordatus and senecio fuchsii have the same, if not even greater strength.

Four parts of goldenrod and one part of juniper berries (or common centaury) make a good, completely harmless drink for good sleep (half an hour before going to bed).

JW: We have different kinds of them. Apart from the ones described by father Künzle, there is a widely spread and still fast spreading newcomer, the Canadian one (solidago canadensis). Most probably it was not here in father Künzle's times. The local variety is much more modest in its looks and in its spreading habits. It is like a country girl in comparison to a film star. Locals trust in the healing power of the local one more, although all varieties of solidago are beautiful and useful.

It is a herb for men as locals believe that it helps for prostate inflammations. But both, men and women use it as a diuretic, as a body cleaning herb and for their kidneys and bladder, for rheumatism and gout as well as for sore throat.

JC: Solidago is the much-maligned Goldenrod. This beautiful plant that paints the rolling hills of old pastures and roadsides in bright yellow where I live in late summer is most often blamed for the nasal allergies caused by the less showy Ragweed (Ambrosia) that blooms about the same time. However, few know that both plants are anti-allergenic! The flowers of the Goldenrod and the leaves of the Ragweed make excellent tinctures and tasty teas to treat the very symptoms caused by pollens. Few pastimes are more enjoyable than sipping a tea of these herbs streamside, while fishing on one of those bright early fall days, when the sun is still hot but the air has just a touch of a chilly nip, and the hills are painted with gold!

Herbal flower hay

is good for extracting abscesses. The wild meadow flower hay is better than cultivated flowers hay, but the flower hay of a nutrient poor meadow, especially the mountain meadow, is the best of wild hay.

Anyone who has 20-40 different kinds of medicinal herbs can simply mix them and get the medicine that is better than any hay. It is quite a mistake when you want to sift them beforehand; for the dust does not consist of feces, but of the decayed very ripe herbs.

If you want the hay to show its full strength, you have to simmer it for at least an hour.

JW: This is something very specific in the Alpine area. People believe in the power of the herbs growing in the untouched alpine meadows. They use the cut hay as a natural painkiller and treatment for sciatica and lumbago, stiff neck or stiffness coming from draft colds, chronic tension, rheumatism, signs of wear and tear on the joints and spine, cramps, colic, kidneys and bladder pains, Inflammation of the female abdominal organs. Also, for colds, bronchitis, whooping cough....

But it is not to be used for heart and circulatory problems and one should not use it if one suffers from hay fever.

Fr. Kneipp used meadow hay for his water procedures.

Herbal hay is still popular, and one can buy readymade linen sacks filled with hay, or, one can prepare hay oneself by mixing different herbal plants, collected in Alpine meadows, filling 2/3 of a linen sack with herbs and sewing it. Be careful not to use

any metal parts for closing the sack, as it is used heated and metal can cause burns on the skin.

For actual use, one moistens the sack a bit and puts it over the steam - over simmering water. It sounds complicated and needs some practice.

One can use a frying pan, put some stones into it, fill the pan with 3 cm of water, bring the water to simmer, place a hay sack on the stones and cover the pan with a lid, while keeping water simmering on a low heat. You heat the sack for about 20 minutes and turn it once. Then take the lid off, take the sack out with a fork or gloves. Be careful. It's hot! Shake it well, so that the warmth can spread, check the warmth with your hand and put it on the painful area. Wait until you are sure that it is not too hot before you cover it with a cotton and a wooden cloth, so that the sack is fully covered. Keep it for 45-90 minutes - as long as it is warm. Weak persons may keep it for 15 minutes. Then stay at least one hour in bed and afterwards wash the area with warm water. The herbs from inside the sack should be thrown away after the procedure, the sack can be washed in high temperatures and used again.

If the pain is in the neck area, fix the sack to the whole area of upper arms, shoulder and neck.
The procedure takes away cramps, relaxes, calms down, increases blood circulation in the area, and releases pain.

JC: This is one of those true German Folk Medicine remedies. Both Saint Hildegard and Fr. Kneipp were great exponents of the Flower Hay treatments. Fr. Kneipp, especially, recommended their use in herbal baths as part of his famous Water Cure. Cold water was his rule, but hot water was allowed when the Hay

Flowers were appropriate.

Hawkweed (Hieracium pilosella)

People who are very weak because of severe blood loss, who are feverish and shivering will recover very quickly if they often get a raw egg sprayed with hawkweed powder.

It grows on stony soil in the Alps; the flower resembles a dandelion in color and in shape, only it is thinner and has a longer, leafless stem and a bitter taste. The cattle like to eat them and then they give a lot of milk; there are many different kinds of the herb, even reddish ones; all have healing power. Hawkweed is also excellent for edema and for all urine buildup.

This wonderful plant will be as effective when boiled in wine, soup or milk.

JW: It grows everywhere. Also in my garden. Our lawn is a natural one with all the wild herbs. We mow it only when grandchildren are round, so that the bees, sitting on the wild flowers do not sting them, when they run round barefoot. Otherwise it is such a fun to watch the herbs in their day and year rhythms. Hawkweed is as persistent as a daisy. No matter how often you cut it or mow it - it is always there. I harvest it before we mow the lawn.

The herb is called Hawkweed, because it makes eyes as sharp as the eyes of hawks. Already Dioscorides and Hildegard von Bingen praised the herb as a means for better eye sight, for sharper eyes. I do not do anything special for better eyesight, but I add this herb to my salad and to herbal infusions. I am enjoying a good eyesight. May be thanks to hawkweed or because I eat a lot of bilberries, carrots. Who knows...

JC: Hawkweed, or "Mouse-ear Hawkweed" is a remarkable herb rarely used today. The Latin name, *Pilosella officinarum*, indicates that it was an official remedy in the Monastic Medicine of the middle ages. Indeed, written accounts show it to be most useful, especially in bronchial complaints. Maude Grieves, writing in her A Modern Herbal in 1935 stated, "None of the Hawkweeds are now much used in herbal treatment, though in many parts of Europe they were formerly employed as a constant medicine in diseases of the lungs, asthma and incipient consumption, but the small Mouse-ear Hawkweed, known commonly as Mouse-ear is still collected and used by herbalists for its medicinal properties." Plants For A Future provides more information regarding the herb's virtues, "Mouse-ear hawkweed relaxes the muscles of the bronchial tubes, stimulates the cough reflex and reduces the production of catarrh. This combination of actions makes the herb effective against all manner of respiratory problems including asthma, wheeziness, whooping cough, bronchitis and other congested and chronic coughs. The herb is mildly astringent, cholagogue, diaphoretic, strongly diuretic, expectorant and tonic. The fresh plant is antibiotic. The plant has been regarded as a specific for whooping cough and is also used in treating other problems of the respiratory system such as asthma, bronchitis and influenza. The herb is also taken in the treatment of enteritis, influenza, pyelitis and cystitis. It is occasionally used externally in the treatment of small wounds and cuts. The plant is harvested in May and June whilst in flower and can be used fresh or dried."

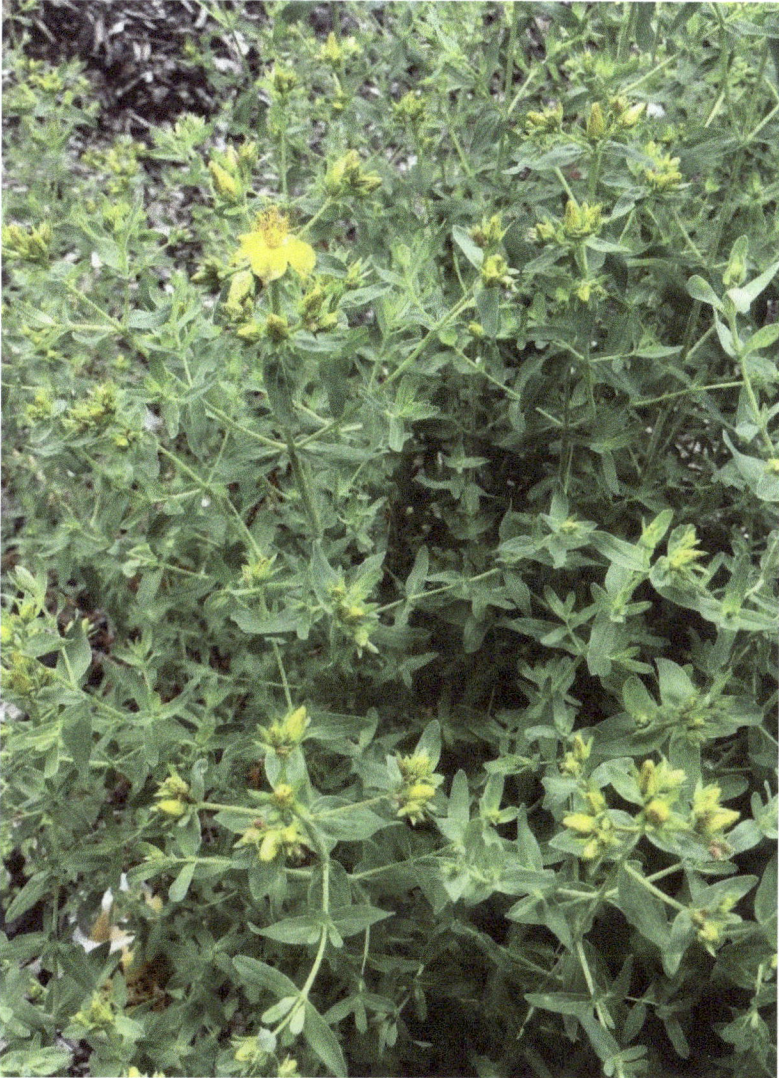

Saint John's Wort

St. John's wort (Hypericum perforatum)

St. John's wort is 30-50 cm high, flowers yellow, each flower has five leaves. In this country you can find three varieties of St John' wort that are very good, and one variety, the largest, which is no good and grows only in swampy places.

St. John's wort can be recognized immediately by the blood. If you squeeze a half-open blossom between your fingernails, blood will come out; the useless variety has no blood. You can find St. John's wort in sunny edges of meadows, on empty farmland, on semi-dry soils, very often in mountainous pastures and in the Alps. The latter are the smallest and have the darkest blood.

The leaves and blossoms of St. John's wort, made into tea, clear the head, clean the mucus from the lungs, stomach, kidneys and bladders; if the infusion is red, take a sip of this tea every hour; it also often helps with blood cramps and abdominal pain.

St John's wort oil is very famous.

This is how you prepare the red oil: take a couple of handfuls of St John's wort flowers, crush them until they bleed, put them in olive oil, put the glass in the sun for ten days until the oil turns red; take as many fresh flowers again, crush them again, put them again in the same oil and again in the sun for ten days; you can do it three to four times until the oil turns dark red.

Use of this oil: It quenches internal and external gangrene in humans and in cattle, it relieves pain from burns and scalds, also from lumbago and rheumatic pain by rubbing it in. It is also used internally for colic; it is used for stab wounds, cuts and bruises and should therefore not be missing in any home.

If the small, well-behaved cat gets a "need", give him a few times St John's wort oil; if an honest, hard-working domestic chicken has symptoms of cough or watery eyes or some inner burn, so that it stands around with its tail hanging, give it some oil.

JW: St John's wort is one of my favorite herbs. Every year I collect the blossoms, every year I try to make red oil. I find the recipe in Father Künzle's book very useful. The red oil is extremely popular in the area where I live. Just like Arnica tincture, you will find St John's wort oil in almost every home.

I like St John's wort infusion. It is my winter evening drink. I like the dark yellow color and a slight odor of honey. No wonder that it has a good reputation among men and women for helping with winter blues, light depression, exhaustion, burn out. The herb is so useful. It is in my mixtures for cold, for digestion, for inner balance and, and, and...

JC: Saint John' Wort is an herb that is certainly in popular use these days. In the 1990s, it received great attention as a useful herb for certain types of depression. Traditionally, it has had many uses, but in the COVID-19 era, many turn to it as an anti-viral. Officially, it is analgesic, antiseptic, antispasmodic, aromatic, astringent, cholagogue (promotes the discharge of bile), digestive, diuretic, expectorant, nervine (calms the nerves), resolvent (helps reduce inflammation), sedative, stimulant, vermifuge (kills parasites) and vulnerary (wound healing). The herb should not be used by pregnant women, however, as it could be dangerous.

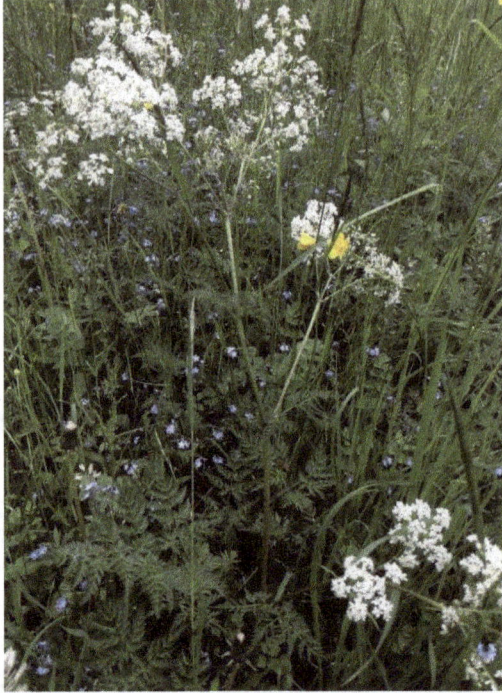
Chervil

Caraway, Anis, Fennel, Chervil, Parsley.

They help with flatulence (bulking in cattle), swelling of the body; all people who only have hard defecation and therefore a pressure in their head, headache, nausea after every meal should take one of these medicinal herbs daily.

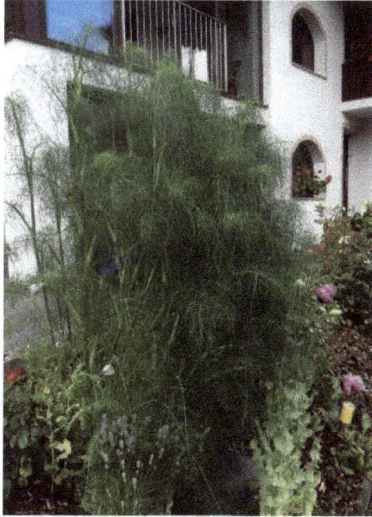

Fennel

One can enjoy them as tea (simmer for a quarter of an hour) or sprinkled as a powder into warm dishes, also boiled with wine or cider. Many people add these herbs pounded in good pomace brandy, leave them there for eight days and strain it. When drinking for pleasure it is usually better to dilute it four to five times.

JW: I would add Dill to this list. It has very similar qualities.

And I have to try Father Künzle's recipe with good pomace brandy as a Digestive. I am sure that is a real treat!

All these herbs are on my spice shelf. I use all of them almost daily. They are in my bread which I bake myself, in my herbal salt, which I mix myself, in salad, in herbal butter... I have frozen dill and parsley in the freezer.

Everybody knows dill - the green leaves of dill, but have you ever tried to use the seeds. Ground seeds. I love this intensive, fresh,

aromatic odor. I put at least a spoonful of ground caraway or dill seeds into a 1 kg bread when I bake one.

My sour cabbage recipe also has a lot of dill or caraway seeds in it. It is an old recipe, and it is logical, that dill is there. Cabbage is notorious for causing flatulence. And caraway and dill are famous for stopping flatulence. So in the end one can enjoy sourkraut without an unpleasant side effect.

JC: My favorite culinary herbs next to the alliums! Our ancestors used these to help with digestion. We also find them in many fermented and preserved foods – pickles, sauerkraut and sausages. No kitchen should be without these simple and very healthful herbs! By the way, parsley is not only good for preventing indigestion, but it is a flavor enhancer that can make most any savory dish taste better... try mixing some parsley leaves into salt, letting them come together for a time and then sprinkling that parsley salt on cheese... it will make very basic cheese, wine and beer taste like the very best!

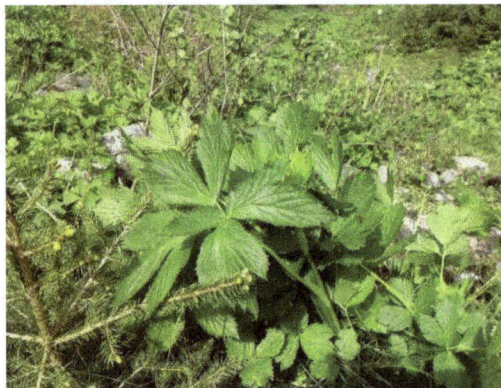

Masterwort

Masterwort (Imperatoria ostrithium)

has been named after the Greek astranthium, and takes its name from the tremendous healing power used by the master healers.

Roots, leaves and seeds are used; autumn is the right time to collect the roots; you can find them in abundance on fertile slopes and between the stones on the Swiss Alps.

Masterwort, boiled and consumed with wine, was considered by the ancients to be the most effective antidote against poison or dog bites. It loosens the mucus from the lungs and is therefore good for those who suffer from severe pulmonary catarrh.

Masterwort, chewed in the mouth, cures the cold in the head very quickly.

Mixed with four parts of salt and well crushed, it cures heavy breathing of the cattle.

Boiled in wine and used as a gargle, it relieves the toothache. The root crushed and applied, eases rheumatic swellings.

Washings with the masterwort water heals eruptions and sores on the head and limbs.

Stomach poisoning from poisonous food is cured by boiling the root in wine and drinking two spoons full every quarter of an hour.

For blood poisoning, mix masterwort powder with water to make a paste and apply as a poultice; it quickly takes the pain away.

Masterwort is one of the herbs having an extracting power; in the case of contagious diseases the ancients carried the herb with them and hung it around the necks of the children.

Those who cannot walk up to the Alps themselves should ask the shepherd to bring masterwort to them, but they have to compensate them for the effort, because the herb clings to the earth like a miser and can only be pulled out by force.

JW: This is a very special herb. A very powerful one! I go up to at least 1800m in the Alps to collect the roots in spring, after the snow is gone or in autumn, which is sometimes in August, as snow can come unexpectedly and early up there.

Once you see the "claws" (the root has sections and if you tear one from the other, you see the "claws", the "fixing part") you know, why grownups and children would carry it - it would protect against all evil spirits. And once you taste the root, you will know - this root kills any germ, virus or fungus.

I slice the washed and cleaned roots, dry them well and have a little bag with roots in my handbag. Whenever I feel the first symptoms of cold, sore throat, cough or anything with digestion or poisoning, I just take one piece into my mouth and keep it as long as whatever is there is gone. I make root tincture for digestion or diluted as mouth water.

One valley in the Austrian Alps is famous for its Masterwort Schnaps. Zillertal! Worth trying.

JC: Masterwort is another herb that should be investigated and utilized more by modern herbalists. Our modern system of food production, storage and sale has resulted in a reduced need for herbs used against "stomach poisoning". However, this is not without cost. While our ancestors employed herbs and

fermentation both for food preservation and to help the body process those foods that were a bit past their prime, we are much weaker in this regard. Yes, our food is "safer" if often less nutritious or flavorful, but those bombarded with antibiotics and pasteurized foods often lack the "Gut flora" necessary to handle even the slightest taint. Such issues need much more thought and often, legislation that could lead us to be a bit less "safe" but more able to handle the natural world as intended. Saint Hildegard recommended Masterwort, taken in wine, for "any type of fever".

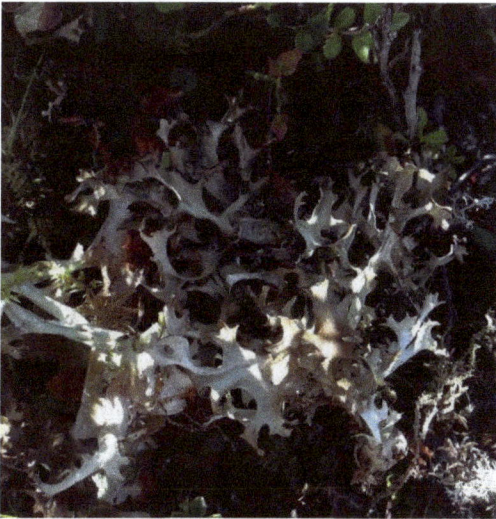

Iceland Moss

Moss (moes)

was used a lot for healing purposes by the ancients. When people and animals were suffering from gangrene and great heat, they would take moss from the stones and place it on the hot spot; you can put cattle on it or tie moss on to them.

Burning feet are also treated with remarkable success.

The common window moss or wreath moss, which is laid between the windows in winter or is used for making wreaths, drives away worms in children when boiled in milk and when taken a few evenings in succession.

Tree moss (the best kind grows on oaks and poplars) boiled with wine or cider cures the strongest diarrhea.

Another disregarded plant created by God for our good!

JW: It is, of course, your decision, whether you will try out any of the Recipes in this book. I did and I feel like sharing my recent experience with moss.

All of a sudden, my husband developed strong back pains. He thinks they came from a sudden and wrong movement. As Father Künzle's remedies is still vividly on my mind I filled a small linen bag with some moss from my garden (ferns which Künzle also advised for usage are not available in early spring) warmed it in the oven, so that it is very warm, but not too hot to put direct onto the skin, placed it on the painful area on the back after fixed it with a woolen scarf. We had in our mind to drive to the countryside and go for a longish walk, but, as it happened, my husband was sure, that we cannot go. In an hour we were in our car, he was driving, and we did walk for an hour or more.

We repeated the procedure the next day twice and my husband was happy to tell me that the pains which developed so suddenly and made walking painful were completely gone.

JC: Moss, like fern, is a category of herb that has fallen a bit out of use. Having written extensively on such herbs as Club Moss

and Usnea, and used them myself, I can attest that they are powerful herbs with many surprising attributes. Various mosses may help the liver or kidneys, strengthen the immune system or help clear the lungs. They are often good for wounds. We need to spend more time in the woods and explore the mosses.

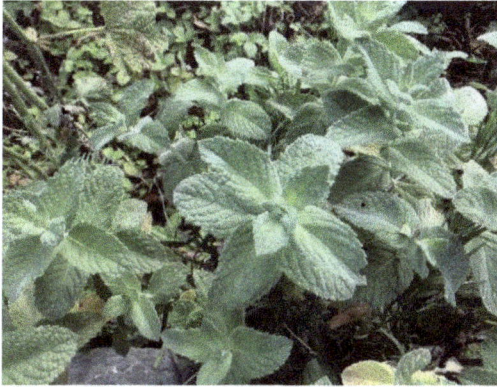

Mint

Peppermint (mentha) or mint

in all their varieties, water mint, wild mint, garden mint, lemon balm, as well as different types of oreganum, marjoram, thyme and wild marjoram reveal their healing power through the aroma. Because of their ability to dissolve entangled substances, excrete diseased substances and entangled gases they are widely used by people and given to cattle. And they increase the healing effect of other herbs.

For headaches, colics and flatulence, take 1-2 cups of very warm tea.

JW: One can use peppermint in so many different ways. I use it as an insect repellent. Just rub it onto my skin. It cools and drives

away mosquitoes. Any mint would do. I use peppermint for Summer drinks. Just a few slices of lemon, peppermint or any other mint, some rose petals, some ground ivy leaves, leave them for 15-20 minutes to soak. It looks nice and it has a gentle flavor from the herbs...

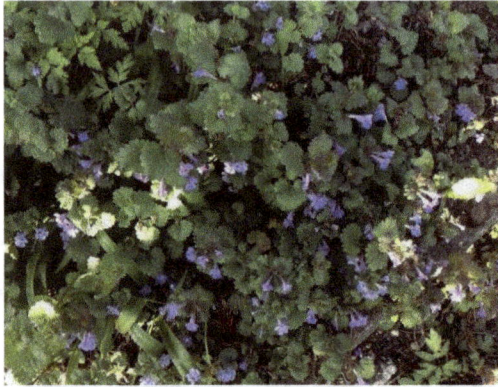

Ground Ivy

JC: I have a particular fondness for the mints.... and not just because I am southern! Yes, the Mint Julep is a stereotypical drink, and surely quite appealing in the right time and place... but I like my bourbon straight. No, for me, mints are the herb of the Blue Ridge Mountains. On most any hike, I can find mint. The variety of the mints that grow here is remarkable. We have all the "usual suspects", the spearmint, peppermint, water mint, etc, but also apple mint and varieties never named. Many summer days, I have wandered these hills and ridges, sustained by grazing on various mints. Medicinally, they are good for a multitude of ailments – from colds and coughs, to digestion and perhaps, even cancer.. and many survivalists chew mint leaves when drinking water from a creek that may be impure, believing the volatile oils will prevent infection.

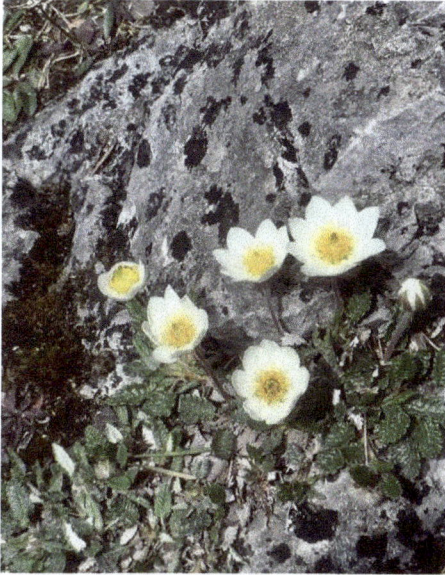

Mountain Avens

St. Benedikt's herb, Wood Avens (Geum reptans, geum urbanum), and all other types of Geum

According to legend St. Benedict gave his blessing to this herb. The best known species of the Geum family - Geum urbanum, also known as Herb Bennet, when dried, smells like finest pinks. Every school teacher knows some variety of this herb, every old dairy farmer knows the best variety of it - the one which grows only high up in the mountains.

The Creator has given St Benedict's herb the power to draw and eliminate everything that should not be in the eyes, nose, teeth, brain nor in the heart; it heals eye ache, headache, toothache, nasal catarrh, also diarrhea, strengthens the heart miraculously and cheers you up.

St. Benedict's herb is one of the plants which can draw out inflammations; probably because of the radium it contains. When the cattle in the Alps get red, inflamed eyes due to the cold wind, the herdsmen tie a bunch of roots of this herb round the neck of a suffering cattle; the inflammation disappears in 1-2 days. I have found out that it works the same with human beings - that eye inflammation and often toothache and headache can be quickly healed with this herb. This power was well known in the past, but now, after it became known that many plants contain radium, the reason for this power has been clarified. The ancients were right again as always.

Fresh roots of St. Benedict's herb, applied fresh and in abundance (do not simmer!) frequently help in case of encephalitis or meningitis or stiff neck. Roots of strawberry plants and tormentil roots have the same effect.

JC: St. Benedict's Herb/Wood Avens is a Rose Family Astringent, often used for maladies of the mouth and throat – sores, ulcers, bleeding gums, sore throat, hoarseness, etc. However, it has many other properties. The herb is anti-inflammatory, antiseptic, diaphoretic and febrifuge (helps to break and control fevers), stomachic (settles the stomach) and styptic. It tightens tissue and is useful for diarrhea irritable bowel syndrome and hemorrhoids. It is even said to reduce or remove freckles. Such herbs are often referred to as YARFAs, Yet Another Rose Family Astringent, because there are many. Just because they are common though, does not mean they are not powerful and extremely useful medicine!

The cranesbill (Geranium robertianum), or Herb Robert.
This plant is mostly used externally, is not exactly poisonous,
but only acceptable to the stomach when mixed with wine; it is
a plant that draws out inflammation. It is a fact, that nasty eye
infections, sore throats, swelling of the teeth, swelling of the
limbs, etc., quickly disappear in people and cattle when green
and crushed cranesbills are applied. If the disease cannot
always be cured by this application, this herb often alleviates
the greatest pain. When dried, it must be soaked in water.

Many other types of geranium, including our well-known
indoor geranium, have the same effect.

The cranesbill is actually famous for healing all types of dry or
wet eczema, eruptions, rashes and sores. In this case, the herb
is boiled and used as a warm bath. In severe cases it is
necessary to continue the treatment for a whole month and
apart from that, drink a spoonful mixed with wine six to eight
times a day!

For the treatment of gastric and mucous fever boil Cranesbill
and let the sick one drink a lot of it; it helps in a day or two.

Fevers are treated with Meadowsweet infusions (Spiraea
ulmaria), or, even better by the white flowers of Hedge
Bindweed (Convolvolus sepium), a well-known weed. The best
remedy for fever is the heart leaved globe daisy (Globularia
cordifolia) – drink a lot of tea of this herb.

The cranesbill is also useful for treating swellings and
inflammations in cattle. Thanks and praise to the Creator!

**JW: This herb is sometimes called "stinking cranesbill". We
use it externally. For something so annoying and always**

returning like herpesvirus. Whenever I start feeling this specific unpleasant itching on the lip... those who develop Herpes from time to time know what I mean, I rub the itching spot with the juice made out of a cranesbill stem and this herpes does not dare to develop any further. But, as I always repeat - we are all different with different immune systems... what works on one, does not necessarily work on somebody else. And cranesbills are different, depending on where they grow, how strong they are.

One could use crushed cranesbill for rashes, eczema. Externally.

JC: Cranesbill has many properties similar to the Rose Family Astringents, it is very astringent and antiseptic. The root is a particularly good treatment for diarrhea and even dysentery, and therefore, good to have on hand as a first aid herb, especially if you have children. Its use against rashes and eczema is not well known; Fr. Künzle has brought us important information!

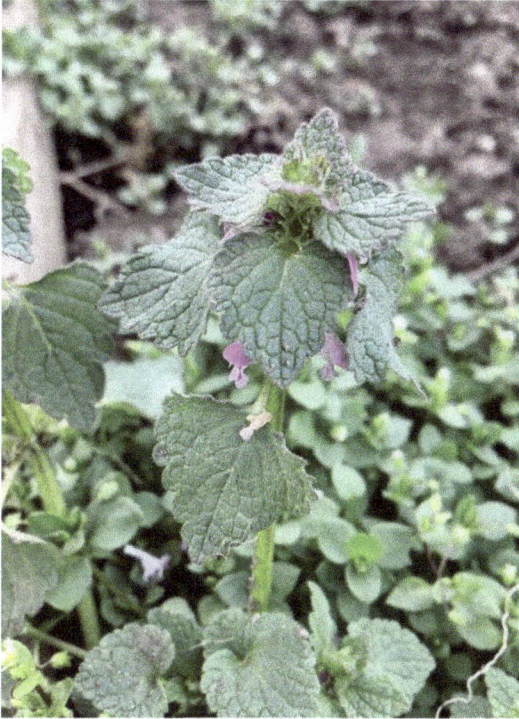

Dead Nettle

The dead nettle (Lamium)

resembles a nettle so much that only experts can tell the two apart, before it begins to blossom. As soon as it blooms, every child can distinguish it; they have flowers around the stem with overhanging roofs; there are white, yellow, red, spotted dead nettles. The white and yellow ones are considered to be the best. The children pluck the blossoms off and suck the honey.

God has given this plant the power to cool, to kill fever, heat and inflammation; it relieves diarrhea in humans and in cattle. Old men suffering from great pains because they cannot urinate find relief after drinking a few cups of this herb.

This tea is also good for cleaning the blood. Boil the herb for 10 to 15 minutes.

Collect the whole plant during the flowering season, and dry it in the sun long and often. When boiled for two hours and left standing, this plant produces a thick jelly which cannot be cut with a knife, as it evades like an eel. This jelly is a wonderful coolant for burns and inflamed feet.
The same tea helps against inflammation in the bladder (recognizable by the red, sharp urine).

JW: As a child I did the same - suck nectar out of dead nettle blossoms. My grandchildren do that and, I am sure that their grandchildren will also enjoy the sweetness of the dead nettle blossoms.

Have you noticed that dead nettles bloom in different colors? Well, different colors mean different stories about how to use them.

Here they say that the red ones are for men. Men, as is indicated in Father Künzle's book, use it for prostate problems. They would collect the blossoming tops of the red nettle and drink infusions.

Women would use the ones with white blossoms against female inflammations and infections. They would make sitting baths. Soaking 5 spoonful's of dried herbs in half a liter of boiling water, keeping it for 10-25 minutes, straining and pouring into a warm sitting bath.
Nowadays it is known that all dead nettles have a very similar effect whether it blooms white, or yellow, or red.

They are used for cold and coughs, help to dissolve mucus, soothe inflammations.
I add fresh herbs to my salads, herbal butter and cottage cheese and to spring body detox infusions.

JC: The Red Dead Nettle grows in my yard, so I was unaware of the many more uses of the White Dead Nettle. Plants For A Future lists the properties of the White as, "an astringent and demulcent herb that is chiefly used as a uterine tonic, to arrest inter-menstrual bleeding and to reduce excessive menstrual flow. It is a traditional treatment for abnormal vaginal discharge and is sometimes taken to relieve painful periods. The flowering tops are antispasmodic, astringent, cholagogue, depurative, diuretic, expectorant, haemostatic, hypnotic, pectoral, resolvent, sedative, styptic, tonic, vasoconstrictor and vulnerary. An infusion is used in the treatment of kidney and bladder complaints, diarrhoea, menstrual problems, bleeding after childbirth, vaginal discharges and prostatitis. Externally, the plant is made into compresses and applied to piles, varicose veins and vaginal discharges. A distilled water from the flowers and leaves makes an excellent and effective eye lotion to relieve ophthalmic conditions." The Red is simply, "astringent, diaphoretic, diuretic, purgative and styptic." Once again, Fr. Künzle has brought us valuable information, in that the herb's use of prostate issues is not well known. Dead Nettle is often considered a weed in America; perhaps the publication of this book will help people realize that it is a wonderful and valuable herb... certainly more so than grass!

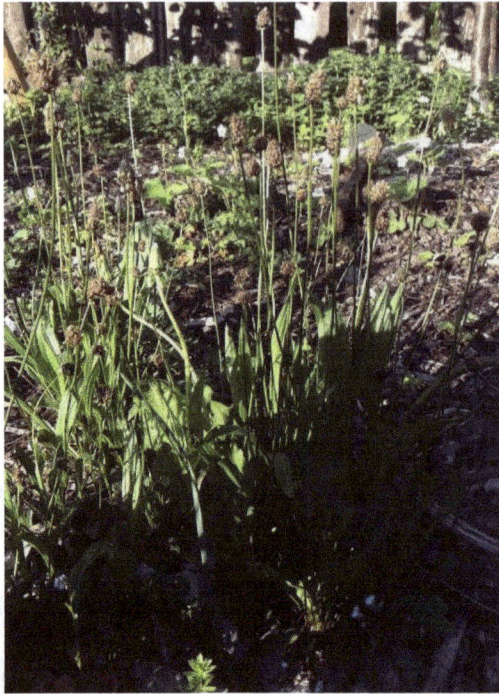

Plantain

Plantain (Plantago) Broadleaf Plantain, Ribwort Plantain

is a very underestimated herb, but it is indisputably the first and the best and most common of all medicinal herbs. God has scattered it on all roads, in all meadows and slopes and it grows in all the climates, so that you always have it at hand.

There are about seven varieties in Switzerland, and all of them have healing power. They are like seven brothers of the same blood. The most common and most underestimated one is the broadleaf plantain (Plantago major); it resembles the poor day laborer who belongs to the lower layers of the society and yet who serves everybody, who cleans the ditches and elects the government, but never gets elected himself. At most one collects the seeds of this plantain as bird food; otherwise it is trampled on by young and old.

Hoary plantain (Plantago media) or a meadow plantain is somewhat weaker in its healing power; it already is a bit more popular, but the farmer does not like it, because it takes up too much space; the farmhand just pulls it out.

Ribwort Plantain (Plantago lanceolata) is doing much better. It is weaker than the previous two, but is already better dressed and is gladly welcomed.

There are four more varieties of plantain that resemble the Ribwort Plantain in the mountain areas; the best and most popular is the Plantago alpina. This is by far the most healing one of all plantain varieties, but it can only be found from 1,800 meters upwards up to the eternal snow.
The best and the most common of all plantains in the valley is the Broadleaf Plantain.

All parts of all kinds of the Plantain are used: roots, leaves, flowers and seeds. It cleans the blood, lungs and stomach like no other herb, so it is good for all people who have anemia, bad blood, weak lungs, a weak voice, pale appearance, with rashes, eruptions, eczema, sores, who cough forever, who have a hoarse voice, stay lean like goats, even if you put them in butter. It helps weak children who fall behind in their development despite of good food.

Preparation. Boil a kettle full of green or dry plantain with 1-2 handfuls of juniper berries or green juniper twigs for three hours in plenty of water, then pour away the herbs and simmer the broth with ordinary sugar for another 2-7 hours. This juice is poured into jars or jugs and stored in the cellar. You can drink as much of it as you want, especially on an empty stomach in the morning. This juice is an excellent remedy for toothache and, by the way, so pleasant that you have to hide it from sweet-toothed children and wasps, but it doesn't last long.

In addition, the plantain in all its varieties helps against toothache (chewed or as an infusion and gargled with it) when applied externally. It also heals wounds and cuts (crushed and applied) as quickly as arnica.

Praise and thanks therefore be to the almighty Creator and Father for giving us such a great remedy in such an abundance!

JW: One can write many stories about Plantain. It is such a useful plant. My first help during hiking. When I have a little wound, a bruise or a blister - I chew a leaf a bit or crush it, so that the juice comes out and put it on the injured place. It stops the bleeding and helps the wound to heal. One can fix it with a band aid so that it stays on a blister in a shoe.

I use it against mosquito bites or nettle stings. Even my grandchildren look for one when they feel a mosquito bite. They just rub an effected area with the crushed leaf and the unpleasant feeling is gone.

For a sore throat I chew a fresh leaf very slowly, so that the mucus from the leaf covers and soothes the sore throat.

The healing mucus in Plantain is easily destroyed by the heat; thus, one should never pour hot water on it. Pour cold water over the cut plantain, leave it during the night to soak, strain the liquid and slightly warm it before drinking.

For winter colds, I make plantain honey: I chop the herb very thinly and place it in a jar in layers with honey or sugar. One is supposed to "bury" this medicine for three months in the ground. Yes, true, in the ground about 50 cm deep where the temperature is low and steady.... or... nowadays one can 'bury' it in the fridge. It is a good medicine for coughs where mucus has to be dissolved.

I add fresh leaves to my salad, I add seeds to my yogurt, soup, muesli...

One could write a novel about a plantain - it is such a useful plant!

JC: It is wonderful how Fr. Künzle's mind worked. He goes immediately from one herb considered to be a weed in American lawns to another, making it easy for us to understand and remember his recommendations. For a man who would have had little concept of an American lawn, and for whom to disregard such powerful herbs would have been almost sacrilegious, it is uncanny how he speaks to us today! Along with the ubiquitous Dandelion, Plantain is perhaps the most common "weed" in this country. But also with the Dandelion, it is excellent medicine. Those who do recognize its properties often use it as first aid for insect bites and stinges, cuts and all manner of abrasions. It is a good pot herb, too, cooked with a little fat and salt, served with vinegar. Even the modern reader who may have no knowledge of herbs, probably knows the seeds of Plantain as Psyllium, the popular laxative. An excellent use for Plantain, Stinging Nettles, Mint, Red Clover and many other herbs is as an infusion – pour hot water over an ounce or more of the herb, let stand and cool overnight. Sipped on throughout the day, these infusions are refreshing, immune supportive, hydrating and an excellent source of vitamins, minerals and the healthy properties of the herbs.

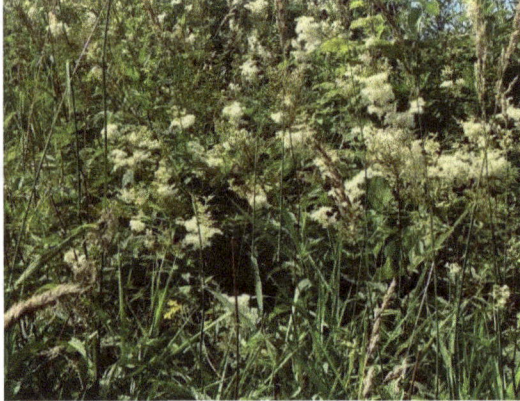

Meadowsweet

Meadowsweet (Filipendula ulmaria)

can be found in all wet places, in ditches and in standing water in huge quantities. This despised herb is a miraculous gift from God because its blossoms are so soothing when used for
1. fever;
2. diarrhea and calf paralysis;
3. Prepared with wine and drunk for edema;
4. Rheumatic ailments of all kinds. (Boil blossoms with wine and drink often!)
5. The leaves work well on stab wounds and cuts.

JW: It is one of my favorite plants. I cannot imagine going through a year without meadowsweet. It became even more famous when Bayer started producing aspirin from meadowsweet and willow bark. Does it ring a bell? If Bayer can make business out of it, why can I not take a Meadowsweet and

willow bark and make my own home medicine without side effects?

Meadowsweet thins the blood. Be careful, if that is an issue!

It is a beautiful herb. The blossoms are like foam or white cotton, the smell is pleasantly sweet with a hint of almond. I collect blossoming tops and sometimes I make my favorite whipped cream: just immerse the blossoms into cream, cover tight, leave them in the fridge for the night, then take the blossoms out and whip the cream. The cream will taste of almonds - the odor of the meadowsweet.

If I have fever or pains in joints - I always add it to my mixtures or make a special mixture of meadowsweet and powdered willow bark. Some make meadowsweet blossom syrup. It tastes delicious.

JC: Meadowsweet was once a very popular medicinal herb that many have forgotten. It was one of the "sacred herbs" of the Druids. The herb is strongly anti-inflammatory and antiseptic. It soothes an upset stomach and is a diaphoretic. Fr. Künzle would not likely have agreed with the Druids on matters of theology, but in that herbs are indeed sacred gifts from God I am sure he would have been in accord. It is likely no coincidence that the Patron Saint of herbalists is Saint Fiacre, who was an Irish abbot, priest and eventually, a religious hermit. Overwhelmed by the crowds of people that flocked to him for his herbal cures, Saint Fiacre took his knowledge and love of gardening from his native Ireland to France, where the famous herbalist could live a quieter life in prayer and contemplation. My heritage being largely both Irish and French, I had to mention that!

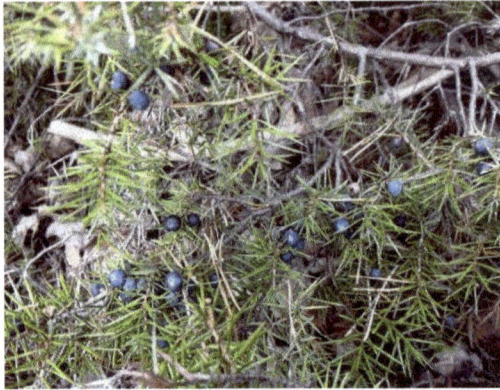

Juniper

The juniper or Reckolder (Juniperus)

is a medicinal plant of the first rank; everything about it is medicinal: wood, needles, berries, bark.
It has the power to warm up, relieve internal colds, cleans everything whatever it can reach, stomach, intestines, lungs, blood, and is therefore used in almost all herbal mixtures, except for hot diseases (such as fever etc.).

Even stronger than the common Juniper is the kind found on the high Alps that creeps along the ground.

Juniper baths are usually a good remedy for old rheumatisms; I have seen old people twisted by gout become straight and healthy again through continued use of such baths; and how people who stayed in bed stiff like a piece of wood for six months were healed by washings and later bathing in Juniper decoction.

Of course, the green Juniper twigs have to be boiled for three hours; the patient is washed with this (warm) water ten times a day all over his body until he is able to take a bath.

Because the bath is very sharp and aggressive, it is advisable to mix it with fir tree or green pine tree twigs' decoction. The baths must be warm and last for half an hour; At the end the whole body has to be poured over with cold water; if you fail to do this, it is better not to take the bath, otherwise the rheumatism will come back even more severely.

JW: Whenever I see a juniper with berries/cones on my walk in the forest, I collect a few junipers ripe - black or dark blue ones and chew them while walking.

I love them: they have a sweetish and a very aromatic taste and I know that they will strengthen my body and spirit.

Fr. Sebastian Kneipp, who has already been mentioned more than once in this book, suggested juniper cone therapy after a long illness, exhaustion, after cancer treatment, etc, because Juniper cones clean the body, clean the blood, improve metabolism. They are good for rheumatism, arthritis, they have an antibacterial effect. Besides, they are tasty, disinfect one's mouth and leave a nice flavor.

Kneipp suggested a 23 days juniper cone therapy. One consumes 213 cones all in all.
On the 1st day one chews and swallows 4 cones;
On the 2nd day – 5...
3rd day – 6
Each day one cone more until one reaches 15 cones on the 12th day.
Then one cone less every day until one reaches 4 on day 23rd which is the last day. And then one should make a long break, so that the kidneys are not harmed. (One should not experiment with this treatment if one has kidney problems).

I myself have never managed to do the full treatment. My way of giving my body a different variety of wild plants includes juniper cones now and then. Powdered, I use them as a spice for meat dishes, and I add juniper to my herbal salt.

I add twigs to inhalation mixtures, to my incense mix, I clean my home with juniper twigs smoke. It is not easy to pick them, however, there is a belief that even staying near or passing by juniper bushes cleans lungs, kills bacteria and viruses. Thus, it is worth collecting a few twigs or cones now and then.

JC: Juniper is also an excellent herb to stimulate appetite and to help the liver. It is a natural bitter, and just thoroughly chewing and eating a few berries before a meal can be among the best helps in digestion for elderly and chronically ill people. Care should be taken not to over use them though, as in large amounts they can irritate the kidneys. Juniper is also good for the immune system and cleaning the blood – a good spring tonic.

Cure with Figs

Around 50% of all illnesses are caused by constipation, as Kneipp stated after thirty years of experience. If the constipation is not cleared, no medicine will work and the problem will return after an apparent cure.

Constipation affects all those people who do not have at least one bowel movement a day, or who always have hard, forced bowel movements.

The gases emitted during bowel movements and winds cause headache, eye pain, etc.; in other people the gases press on the chest, on the stomach, abdomen; these people then always complain that they are so full or anxious.

The simplest, most harmless means for good stool movement is the fig cure, applied for one to two months. How do you do the fig cure?

Take 5 to 10 common figs every evening, wash them in lukewarm water, then put them in a glass and pour cold water onto them until they are covered; in the morning eat all the figs on an empty stomach and drink the water that is still in the glass.

The cure is much more effective if you cut the figs and soak them in olive oil for a day; Instead of figs, you can also use dry pears or dry plums in the same way.

The figs as you know are full of small grains; these gradually remove the mucus from the stomach and intestines, whereupon the stomach and intestinal skin are free and clean and can work properly again. If you gradually get too much bowel movements, i.e. more than three times a day, stop the fig cure for the time being. The figs can be finely chopped for small children. Those who suffer from hard stools, beware of chocolate and cocoa, they are like the plague to you.
Dried pears, dried plums, dried apricots, soaked in water for a day, eaten on empty stomach in the evening before bedtime, have the same effect.

JC: I certainly do need encouragement to eat figs – they are one of my favorite fruits! A good fig is a delicacy on its own, but you may also enjoy trying them with honey, nuts, blue cheese or ham. Additionally, the leaves are medicinal, being used as a tea to settle the stomach and in baths for various inflammations.

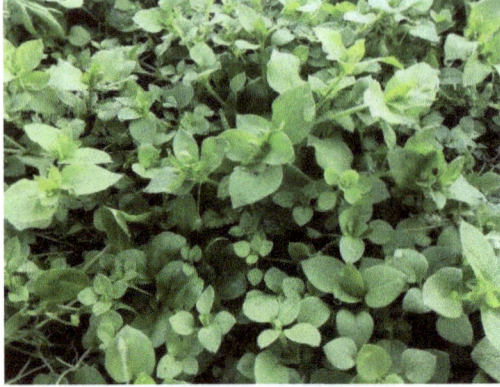

Chickweed

Chickweed (Stellaria Media),

If you have a canary bird, you put plenty of this herb in its cage; other birds like it too.
To humans, these weeds, which overgrow entire patches, are priceless. It is a wonderful tool for strengthening the heart, brings back strength and freshness to people who have been ill for a long time; but do not dry these little herbs, because like vegetables they would otherwise lose their strength; you can prepare it like spinach with a little flour and meat stock, or boil it and drink the juice.

Its juice is also excellent for children's gout. Even tuberculosis patients have been cured after prolonged use of this divine gift of God.

Externally, the crushed herb is applied as poultice for pneumonia, liver inflammation, throat swelling, inflamed feet, rectum, etc.

All related varieties that the botanist finds in the Stellaria and

Cerastium families can also be used in the same way; the alpine varieties are even more powerful.

JW: I could not agree more to what Father Künzle wrote about chickweed. It is a very useful and delicious herb (I cannot call it a weed) and I eat it almost daily during the spring months. When other herbs appear, chickweed goes into compost or food for birds.

I add a lot to salad, to spice butter, spice curd, it makes omelets taste better. I like it. It tastes a bit like nuts or like peas.

And it is good for the health! Chickweed has 10 times more Vitamin A and C than Salad. It is rich in Potassium, Calcium, Magnesium. 150 grams of Chickweed covers the daily need of Iron, Potassium and Vitamin C. It also contains Saponins, this foaming ingredient and helps with Bronchitis. Saponins also protect the stomach lining and intestines lining.

It is still used locally for soothing the pain of Rheuma, Arthritis and Gout (cut or beat the chickweed until juice comes out and put it on the sore place). Or for soothing a mosquito sting by rubbing chickweed into the skin.

Chickweed multiplies very quickly. That is the reason why it is not so popular among gardeners. One plant can spread up to 15 000 seeds. Thus, the more we eat or use as a home medicine, the fewer we have to weed out.

JC: Chickweed is a wonderful herb that tastes somewhat like spinach. It is a green that will be among the first to appear in the spring. Chickweed, applied topically or added to a bath is good for itchy skin and inflammations. It is good to use as a poultice on sores. A tea made of chickweed is good for kidney issues. It is another of our under-valued "weeds".

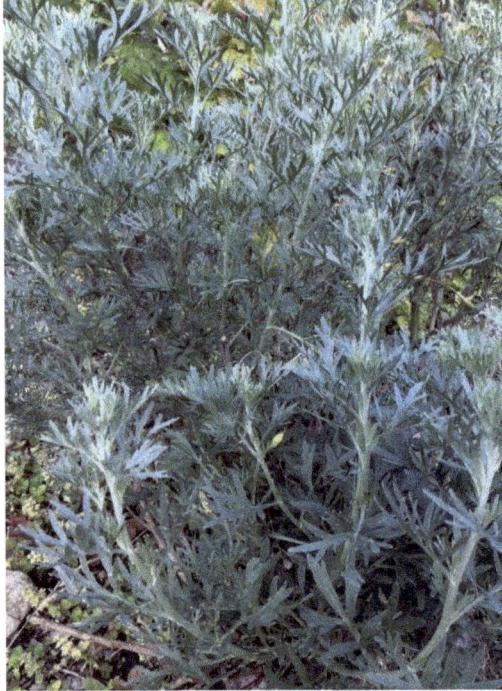

Wormwood

Wormwood (Artemisia, Absinthum), Wormet.

In all its varieties, wormwood is medicinal. Whether infused in water or boiled in wine, it is so strong that one should only take a teaspoon at a time; six to eight teaspoons a day is enough. It helps with a weak stomach, poor digestion, lack of appetite, against anemia and jaundice and drives away worms (hence the name Wormwood).

If one is as green as a tree frog, as thin as a poplar, loses weight and humor every day and no longer casts a shadow, then he should try a teaspoon full of wormwood every two hours; however, wormwood is not to be mixed with any sugar. (Sorry, sweet tooth!)

It helps people suffering from a lot of bile. An old pagan doctor wrote 2000 years ago: "Wormwood is a good medicine for evil, bile-driven women who constantly soak their bodies with overflowing bile and thereby bring different sufferings to many".

Wormwood boiled in wine and drunk quite warm, helps immediately by griping pains and colic and is often effective against edema when used for a longer time. Painters should drink 1-2 teaspoons of wormwood a day, as this medicine expels the white lead.

Externally, wormwood is used against scabs, eczema, eruptions on the face and on the body of people and on cattle. Wormwood is boiled in vinegar; it is used for washing and for making poultices. Poultices put on the forehead and before going to bed bring sleep to nervous people and to those who suffer from insomnia.

Wormwood, well boiled in water and strained heals red, tarnished, weak eyes.
Bitter wormwood is just as healthy for the body as is the poisonous bile for the mind. So plant now a wormwood for me in your garden and thank Him who created it for you to heal!
An intern writes to me: I use wormwood tea, not only for the stomach, but also for cleaning the lungs and combined with sage I use it in order to remove noxious juices and diseased substances from the body. However, I rarely use it in cups, only to achieve a momentary forceful effect, but as a rule by the spoonful, i.e. two spoons full or one sip every half hour.

JW: It is a very popular herb even nowadays and many would have it in their gardens. The locals take it as a good help for digestion. Especially after eating some heavy, fat meal. It is also an ingredient in bitter mixtures - a mixture of bitter herbs used before a meal for better digestion and for a low appetite. It is said to decrease craving for sweet products and sugar. Thus it is very popular among those, who want to lose weight.

Some believe that it helps with constipation, although I would prefer a cure with figs.
Wormwood has been used in different spirits like vermouth (the German name for wormwood is Wermut) or Absinth (the Latin name is absinthium). Well, it is strongly established in our gardens and homes.

I have linen sacks filled with wormwood in my wardrobes. Against moths and other insects. And I grow it in my kitchen garden as I believe that it helps keeping plants safe from insects.

JC: Wormwood is one of the most important and ancient medicinal herbs known to man. Many American readers may actually recognize the old German name of the herb that came to be pronounced in more modern times as "vermouth". Yes, the common herbed wine that is famous for being an ingredient in the martini, was originally made with wormwood!
Wormwood has been included in many famous wines and liquors. The absinthe (over) enjoyed by many artists was in part, a very highly alcoholic Wormwood liquor. Wormwood is a great bitter, that stimulates digestion, the liver and gallbladder. It helps relieve flatulence. It helps with blood sugar. Officially, it is "anthelmintic, anti-inflammatory, antiseptic, antispasmodic, antitumor, carminative, cholagogue, emmenagogue, febrifuge, hypnotic, stimulant, stomachic, tonic and vermifuge." And yes, it contains thujone... which, in large amounts is intoxicating.

However, that amount is so large that many of the artists who went insane probably did so due to drinking large amounts of 150 proof alcohol! Still though, caution should be used. Most instances of toxicity trace to people trying to make their own absinthe with essential oil of Wormwood, which is extremely poisonous.

Spring cure

There are many people who, without being bedridden, are almost always unwell, they have no appetite and dislike the best St. Gallen sausages, are clogged up like the gates of hell, they feel pressure on their chests and in their stomachs and there is heat and pain in the head. They can not sleep well and when they do sleep then restlessly and they have bad dreams; they run after all doctors and are a nuisance to them, write to all quacks as far as to London and New York, swing like party leaders after an election victory, and are like complaining organs with 365 stops, often with an accompaniment of an orchestra.

If such people have the serious will to get well, they should take one of the so-called spring cures for 8-14 days.

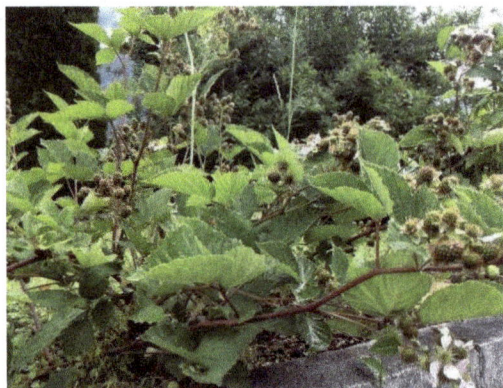

Unripe Blackberries

You send Tony or Jacob into the nearest bushes with a basket and a knife. There he cuts many shoots from all types of thorny bushes: dog rose (Rosa cantina), blackthorn (Prunus spinosa), hawthorn (Crataegus), raspberry (rubus idaeus), and blackberry (rubus fruticosus) and shoots from fir trees, beeches (fagus), hazel trees, cherry trees, oaks, larches, ash trees, poplars. Furthermore you can also take shoots from currants, from gooseberries, from fruit trees.

A handful of this mixture is then thrown into a pan, one to two liters of water are poured in, and the mixture is heated until it simmers. The sick person should drink one to two liters of this liquid daily with sugar. This tea cleanses the whole body. It has already turned very sick people into healthy and flourishing ones again. However, if the effect is to be lasting, this cure must be continued for eight days. The lost appetite returns, the headache and pressure in the abdomen are gone, the pale color vanishes, the grave digger can put his shovel back in his shed. And this poor creature, previously so pale and shaky, can again rule in the kitchen with power and dignity. If she takes five or seven good fir tree twigs baths, she is fresh and sunny again like a bride!

It is known that mustard has extracting qualities, that is why mustard plasters are often used for painful rheumatic areas. The well-known, expensive American plasters contain extracting substances.

The meadow buttercup (Ranunculus acer) is also known to the herdsmen because of its extracting power; if a cow lies down to rest with its udder on buttercups the udder swells up quickly. The buttercup is therefore used like an extracting plaster; but never drink anything with buttercup. It is poison!

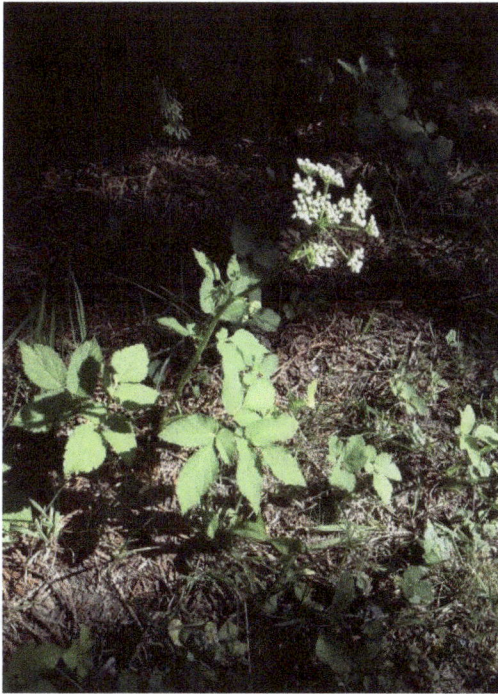

Ground Elder

All plants with sharp juices such as garlic, onion, Alpine leek (Allium victorialis), Cyclamen, raw potatoes, ground elder

(Aegopodium podagraria), Masterwort (Peucedanum ostruthium), have extracting power.

If pain arises anywhere without any visible abscess, as in toothache, earache, in the joints, put one of the bulbs or roots of the above mentioned herbs, raw or squeezed, on the painful area, and in many cases the pain disappears after a few hours; I know cases where a terribly aching ear or a very sore throat was quickly cured in this way. Freshly cut chives have helped often too.

If you carry the well-known Masterwort root with you, it will remove all kinds of disease substances in you. All sorts of illnesses occur in stables, despite all the cleanliness, a basket full of Masterwort put in the stables would soon help to alleviate all these diseases. The root of Pimpinella has the same extracting power.

So the good Lord has surrounded us everywhere with remedies and gave healing power to herbs, blossoms, fruits and to roots.

JW: There are so many pleasant recipes for spring cure. One of my favourite ones is a dandelion blossom cure: every day for a fortnight I take a dandelion flower - not completely open, together with a stem, chew it slowly at least twenty times and swallow it.

Or I have a handful of dandelion leaves with my lunch for a few weeks.

For spring detox and cleansing teas I combine dandelion leaves and roots with birch leaves, dog rose hips, and a bit of peppermint for a better taste. I take a teaspoon of this mixture per cup of tea and drink at least two cups a day for 4 to 6 weeks mornings and afternoons. Not in the evening as it is a diuretic.

When I say, I take it 4 to 6 weeks, that is not very true. I start and then forget. Then start again. The body doesn't mind as long as it is healthy. Or I just add spring herbs to different dishes in different forms and then my food is my spring cure.

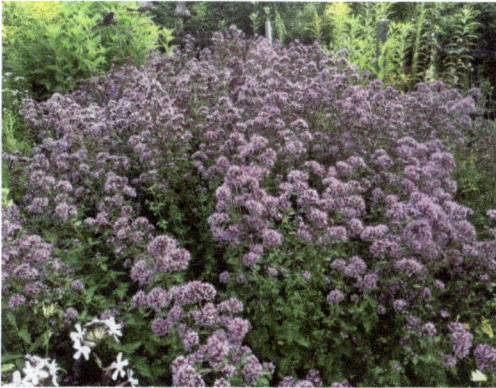

Oregano

Here is my recipe for herb butter:
Ingredients: 250 grams soft butter, 20 grams (or more... the taste will be richer) young herbs: young leaves of goutweed, dandelion, yarrow, garlic, lovage; shoot tips of thyme, oregano, nettle; flowers and leaves of daisies, ground ivy...
Preparation: Wash herbs (not necessary, if you collect them from your own garden), chop finely, puree in very soft butter, season to taste with salt.
If you want a little stronger butter, you can add some cloves of garlic, ground papaya seeds, turmeric and nettle seeds.
Place the butter in the refrigerator for at least one hour and enjoy it!

JC: Here we have many bitter, sour and astringent herbs, along with the aliums. This spring cure would certainly be a good tonic. This would tone the entire system, stimulate the liver and gallblzadder. Several herbs are astringent and others expectorant. Several are cleansing and immune supportive. The Aliums are antiseptic. There are many good vitamins and minerals here, too. I would, however, give caution in regard to the Buttercup, Ranunculus. This is an extremely caustic, irritating, blistering plant. I would prefer to use Mustard.

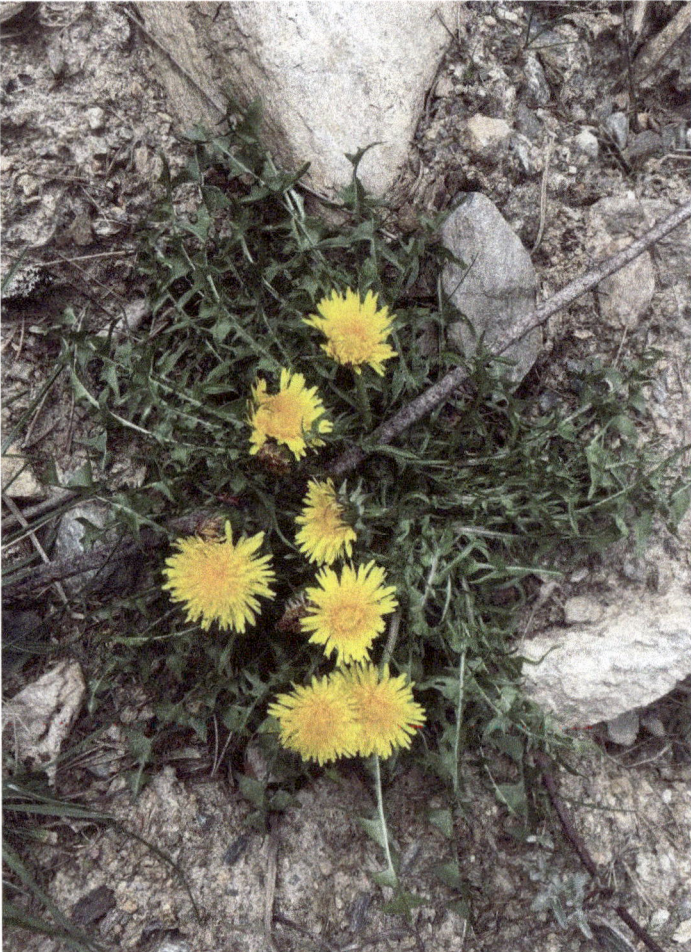

Dandelion

Medicinal spring herbs.

Dandelion (Taraxacum officinale), is dug out avidly by Italians and they prepare and eat it as salad. When boiled and drunk dandelion cleans the blood and loosens gallstones, but one should follow such a cure for three to four weeks.

Sweet violet (Viola odorata) is a wonderful remedy for whooping cough; one also uses young leaves.

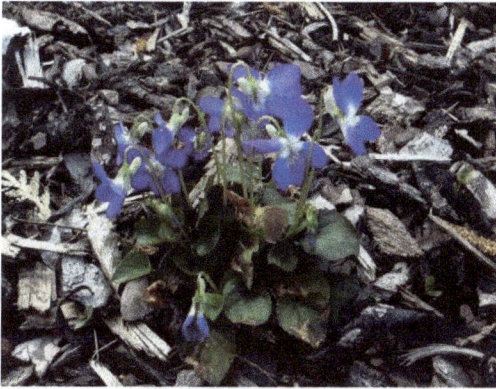

Sweet Violet

Cowslip (Primula **veris**), make a tender, fragrant tea; all varieties of Primula have healing qualities; even better, however, are the dark yellow, fragrant ones; the very best, however, grow in the Alps.
It is drunk as tea; much better, however, when they are boiled in wine and drunk in the evening before going to bed. Kneipp praises them against gout, rheumatism, stiffness in the limbs, but it helps only if used for a long time.

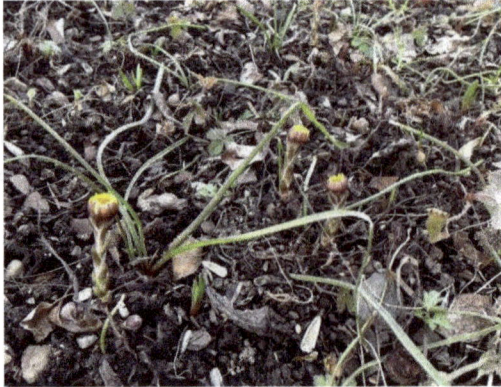

Coltsfoot

Coltsfoot (Tussilago farfara) is almost the first flower to show its yellow head in spring along brooks and in loamy soil. These little flowers together with cowslips are mainly used against cough.

Even more valuable are the large leaves of Butterbur (Petasites hybridus) they are gray below, green above, huge, in the Alps they look like an umbrella; inwardly they are excellent against coughs; they should be dried long and carefully in the sun.

Outwardly, the large leaves are invaluable against any kind of burns, tired feet, infected wounds and swellings, when crushed and applied. The dried leaves are softened in the water.
In case of severe sprains and dislocations, apply a handful immediately.

How many herbs God has sown! Glory and thanks to him!

JW: No wonder that Italians consumed a lot of dandelions a hundred or more years ago. Italian kitchen is considered to be one of the healthiest kitchens and by adding dandelion to the food one does a good favour to one's health. Dandelion leaves contain a lot of Potassium, Iron, Calcium, Magnesium, Vitamins

A, B1, B2, C. Roots contain taraxin, inulin. By adding dandelion leaves, blossoms, roots to one's meals or drinking dandelion infusions, one detoxifies and strengthens one's body. Potassium in dandelion has a very important role in detox teas, as it replaces the Potassium, which is expelled from the body with urine. This is how the body cleans itself, gets rid of toxins and other harmful substances helping also those, suffering from rheumatism and arthritis. One needs to drink a lot alongside with dandelion infusion.

I add loads of spring herbs to my salad. Do you also find salad from supermarkets boring and not nutritious enough? If yes, here is my recipe of salad with wild plants:

If you have a garden, no matter how big or small, there are always good old weeds there or you can bring some from the walks: dandelions- I use young leaves; yarrow - young leaves look like perfect eyebrows; cowslip leaves and blossoms, daisy leaves and blossoms; coltsfoot blossoms, young ground elder leaves, garden cress; leaves of pilewort (Ficaria verna); wood betony tops; chickweed plants...

If you find a nice field during your weekly walks, you can collect fresh herbs from there. The herbs will keep fresh for up to one week if you keep them in a tightly closed plastic bag with some air inside, like a kind of a half inflated balloon. Keep it in the fridge and you will enjoy fresh herbs all week.

We do need Salad. We need a lot of greens, we need chlorophyll, we need fibres, we need vitamins and minerals. They clean our body and blood, help to get rid of cholesterol, strengthen our immune system, keep our heart strong, save us from getting diabetes, cancer...

Can the salad from the supermarkets give us all that?

Salad from the supermarket is like a basic tune in music, to turn it into Jazz you have to add variations and colour.

One does not have to be too creative with the dressing. The herbs will provide the taste. Just add a little bit of olive oil, some home made or natural apple vinegar, some herbal salt... The salad will taste wonderful with some home made bread and herbal butter.

JC: Here, we find that greatest of all weeds, the dandelion. Dandelion is good for the liver, gallbladder, stomach, kidneys... it is a blood purifier and tonic to the entire system. It is also deliscious! Violet is a blood tonic, good for fevers and stregthening to the lungs. Cowslip, among its other medicinal properties, is sedative and relaxing, while helping reduce pain due to its aspirin-like properties. Coltsfoot is particularly good for the lungs and bronchial congestion. Butterbur reduces pain and muscle spasms, supports heart and lung function and is diuretic.

Herbs and weeds

Why did the good Lord create so many weeds so that one is always plagued with weeding? Certainly not because of the intention to torture us; all weeds are medicinal herbs. The good Lord has scattered them everywhere we go, so that whether we like it or not, they are always at hand. Even cats and dogs know this and eat grass from time to time. An old blacksmith advised a pale looking woman - always ill, but not yet dying, to watch her gray cat, because the cat definitely knows the cure. The woman watched her pet, collected the same grass that it ate, boiled it and drank it for some time and recovered completely. What kind of grass is that? Cat grass (Dactylis glomerata) and Couch grass (Agropyrum repens); both are weeds, but for 2000 years doctors regarded them as excellent means for cleaning kidneys and bladder and against all ailments because of urinary problems.

An old herbal doctor prescribed a man suffering from constipation to collect a handful of common meadow grass every day, simmer it and drink it, and it helped.

Bindweeds (convolvus species) are really hated as weeds. They cannot be extirpated, their roots go all the way down to hell and the plant always grows again, entwines all the vegetables and tears them to the ground. But precisely this Bindweed is a wonderful means for fever and quenches all internal inflammations (e.g. soak in water).

In spring many fields are completely covered with chickweed (Stellaria media) as if covered with a green carpet. In May, often already in April, everything is covered with small stary blossoms. This herb keeps moisture in the soil and prevents it from evaporation. Crushed and placed on wounds it takes the heat away and, when drunk as tea, heals fever.

Other fields are covered with the strong and spicy smelling field mint (Mentha arvensis). These weeds are priceless for humans and livestock, they dissolve all internal ulcers, accumulation of mucus, etc., and should be collected in large quantities by all ranchers. When it is not clear what is wrong with the animals, give them mint water for three days, then dried nettles with juniper berries, and the animals will quickly recover.

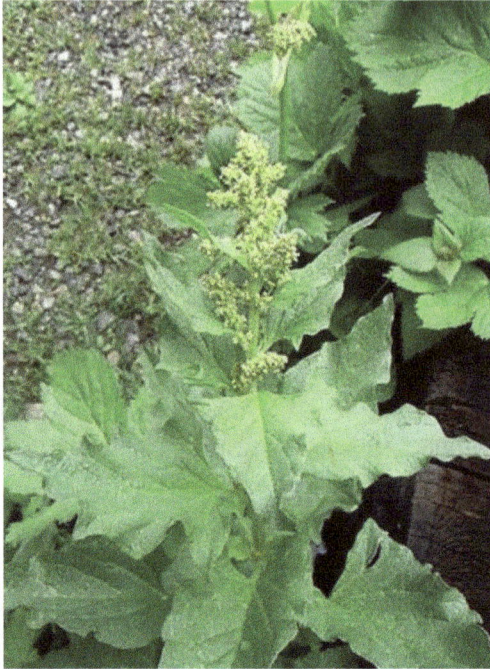

Orache

Garden orache (Atriplex hortensis), a meter-high plant with many side stems, looking like a bushy fir tree and having a colour of a gray cat, is weeded and hated. Those who have a good stomach can boil it and drink it. It helps constipated sinners and constipated cattle quickly and powerfully to get rid of constipation. You can boil it and drink it, but it is better to mix the decoction half half with wine.

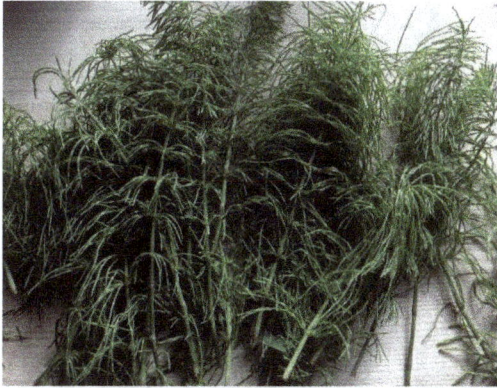
Horsetail

Common groundsel (Senecio vulgaris) with many yellow flowers is also considered to be a useless weed. Crushed and placed on wounds, however, it heals wasp stings, burns and ulcers. Horsetail (Equisetum species) thrives in some fields and one cannot get rid of it; it has often been condemned and angry perpetrators have evoked ghosts! But some of them have already long been resting in the graveyard. If he had collected the horsetail in good time, dried it and used it, he would still be alive and perhaps still grow as old as the Rabbi from Bascher, who would not make his last will before he has seen the Falknis mountain green in summer and white in winter for ninety times.

Pastor Kneipp called the herb "Zinnkraut" and prescribed it for external use against all the rotting wounds, or sitting over steam, against suffering from stones; I have seen for myself how an 86-year-old man recovered from the most terrible suffering from stones after a single steam remedy session and then afterwards he lived for many more years. The horsetail heals the strongest blood flow and Hematemesis taken as tea in a very short time, almost instantly.

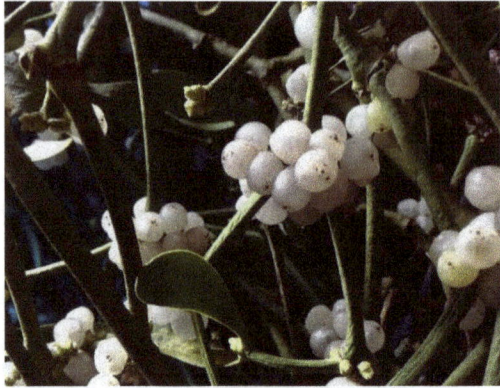

Mistletoe

Mistletoe (Viscum album), is considered to be an annoying, officially and legally forbidden weed that has been eradicated by all municipal councils and country hunters in all 22 departments in Switzerland and despite all the attempts it is still there. Pastor Kneipp says that he can only strongly recommend this weed to all women; a single cup of boiled mistletoe clears blood flow disorders. Thus, in the form of despised and scorned weeds, God has lovingly and with care and as a precaution placed wonderful remedies on the path, into the hands and under the feet of beloved people.

Nothing in nature just happens
Everything is destined from above.
So never blame in ignorance,
What you have not thoroughly understood;
What you fight as your enemy
Often is your very best friend.

JW: I cannot agree more when I read what Father Künzle wrote about herbs and weeds. I use the book for learning more so that I can integrate more herbs into my kitchen and herbal teas. I

have to find out more about bindweed, garden orache or common groundsel.

Horsetail is already firmly established in my home and garden. The dried powdered herb is on my dining table and I take half a teaspoon after every meal for cleaning my teeth and not only for that. It strengthens hair, nails, bones...

It is my favourite fertiliser for my vegetables, flowers and herbs. This reminds me again and again, that I am part of nature. It strengthens not only my body, but also the bodies of my plants. I make a decoction or soak horsetail together with stinging nettle and comfrey before I water my plants with a diluted solution.

I highly respect mistletoe. It is a very special plant.

It is a semi-parasitic shrub as it derives mineral salts and water from the host plant, but, as it is green, it photosynthesises and transpires itself. One can see mistletoes best in winter when the leaves of the trees are gone, as it is green all year round, usually high up on different types of trees. The older the mistletoe, the more round is its form and thus it is more powerful.
Historically the plant played an important role in Druidic mythology. Mistletoe had a reputation of being a remedy for all the illnesses. Celts and Gauls called it „all-heal".

The medicinal value depends partly upon the host plant. The most valuable Mistletoes are from oaks, limes, poplars, ash trees. The less valuable ones are from pines, apple trees.

The plant is known to be good for regulating blood pressure, stimulating the heart, treating arteriosclerosis. It is also used for

treating cancer, especially the negative side effects of chemotherapy and radiotherapy. It boosts the immune system, strengthens the body.
It is also a sedative and is used to ease anxiety and as a sleep aid. Externally infusions and tinctures are used against rheumatism, sciatica.

One uses the leaves and the stems. Not the berries. The plant is slightly toxic, especially the berries. It contains Viscotoxin. The slightly toxic ingredients do not dissolve in cold water; that is why one should make cold infusions: 2 teaspoons of dried leaves and stems per 200 ml COLD water. Leave it for 6-8 hours. This infusion can be used internally and externally. I use it for boosting my immune system.

For external use one can also make a mistletoe tincture. I make it this way: I fill 1/3 of a jar with dried herbs and cover the jar completely with 40% - 60% alcohol. Leave it at room temperature for 14 days, shake daily, filter it and then I have medicine for rheumatism or sciatic pain or any other pain in the muscles or joints.

JC: First, the helpful piest lists the grasses... Cat Grass, which is thought to be good to use in treating tumors, kidney and bladder problems.... then Couch Grass, which is used for kidney, liver and urinary problems. Then, the bindweed.... interestingly, the Field Bindweed has recently shown promise as a powerful medicine against cancer. Orach is a spring tonic that stimulates metabolism and helps the lungs. Groundsel expels worms, helps with fevers and protects against scurvy. The Zinnkraut is the Horsetail plant, equisetum. It is an ancient and unique family of plants, that are very strengthening to the system due to high concentration of minerals. They are good for wounds, skin, teeth, kidney, bladder, etc. The Mistletoe mentioned here is the

European Mistletoe, which is a very good medicine. The American Mistletoe is extremely poisonous and must never be mistaken for the European version.

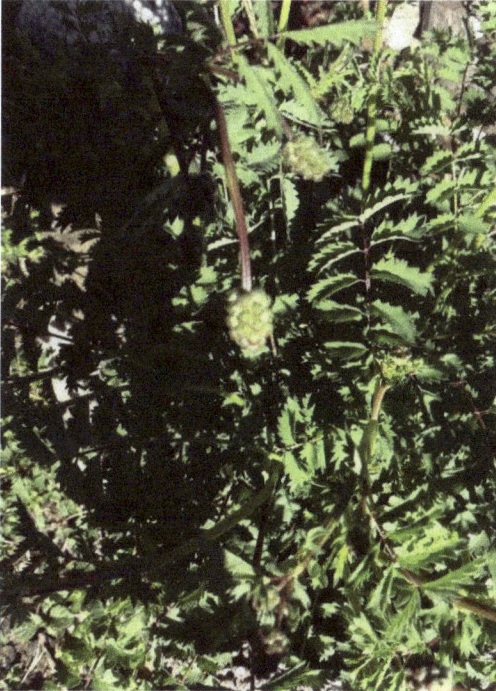

Great Burnet

Hemostatic

The following herbs help with stomach, lung and other bleeding, used as tea (boil thoroughly): the hemostatic agent Great Burnet (Sanguisorba officinalis), especially the root, the large and the small Globularia (Globularia major and minor), both alpine herbs , Eightpetal mountain-avens (Dryas octopetala) are to be found in the High Alps.

JC: Great Burnet is a strongly astringent herb. Globularia is antirheumatic and laxative, mildly stimulant. Dryas is also a strongly astringent that helps settle the stomach.

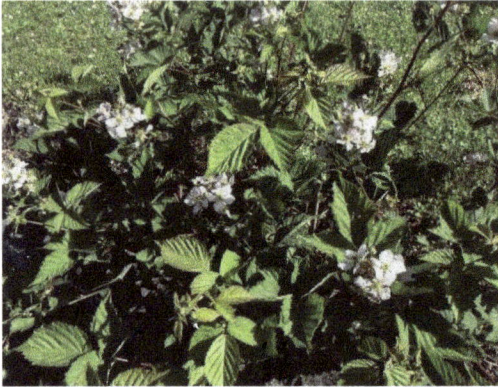

Blackberry

Remedies for diarrhea. (Diarrhea in humans and livestock)

Tree moss (pseudevernia furfuracea), boiled and to be drunk. Common box (buxus sempervirens) - the one that grows in gardens, boiled and to be drunk. Green Blackberry leaves, boiled and drunk, young thicket creeper (Parthenocissus inserta) leaves, hazelnut leaves, green, boiled and to be drunk.

 If you are able to eat them raw, you can eat hazelnut or blackberry leaves or young thicket creeper leaves with bread without boiling them, which can sometimes be useful when you are travelling.

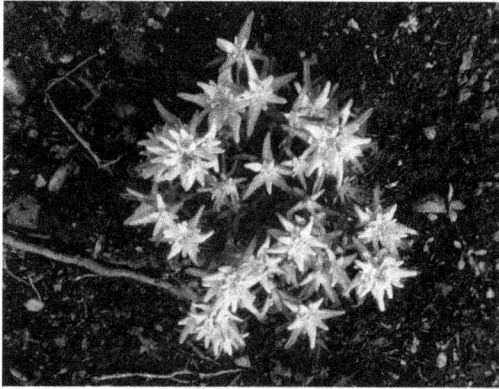

Edeweiss

A good remedy for diarrhea is Edelweiss (4 - 5 flowers are enough) and the related herb Cudweeds (Gnaphalium in all its varieties). Boil these flowers well and drink a cup or two, and the malady is gone. It is even more effective with wine.

Another remedy is the cotton-grass (Eriophorum species) growing in marshes, it has a crown of fine, white wool; boil it and to be drunk.

My best remedy is Tormentill (Potentilla tormentilla). It is to be boiled in wine and to be drunk.

JW: Tormentil is known and used by many for diarrhea, because of the astringent qualities of its root. In German speaking countries it has another name - Blutwurz, which is translated into "bloodroot". It stops bleeding as efficiently as it stops diarrhea.

The local recipe for diarrhea is as follows: pour a cup of cold water over a teaspoon of ground root, bring it to a boil, strain and drink it 3-4 times a day before the meal. Do not add any sugar.

The diluted tincture is used for washing wounds or not diluted for treating inflammations or wounds in the mouth area. It is a powerful herb, thus, not recommended for pregnant women and small children.

JC: What more can be said? The herbs do as he stated. I would include Oak bark.

The chicory (cichorium intybus)

The chicory was already known as a medicinal plant in ancient times. A coffee drink was made from the root of the grafted chicory. So it is by no means a modern factory product, but a herb and a luxury product that has been known for centuries, which was also used to keep the body healthy.

Not only the roots but also the leaves of the grafted chicory are used. Through the roasting process, the root provides the well-known luxury food that we know under the name "chicory" and that has developed into an excellent coffee additive. Chicory owes its wide distribution mainly to its health-promoting properties. In particular, it stimulates the appetite and has a beneficial effect on digestion.

JW:
Chicory is still being used as a coffee drink, even though real coffee is easily available. And many use it for stimulating appetite and digestion.

JC: Chicory comes in multiple forms. There is the pretty little, blue, dandelion type flower and then the endive.... and a few variations of those. It is a good, bitter, tonic herb. It is also a nice bitter salad green. The best chicory infused coffee I have found comes from just a few small companies in Louisiana. Bad chicory coffee is bitter and unpleasant. Good chicory coffee is bitter-sweet, like chocolate. That flavor is enhanced by cream and a shot of bourbon. Made right, Creole coffee is a masterpiece, naturally sweet without the addition of any sugar!

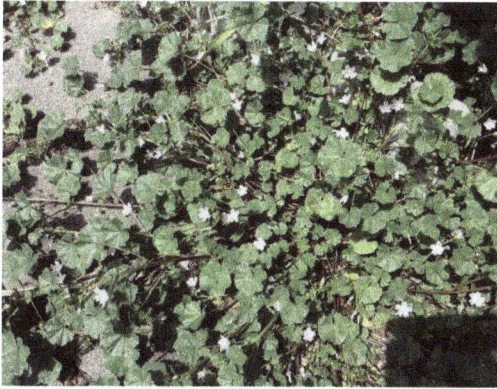

Mallow

Abscesses from the summer heat

Without an animal bite, without any wound or poisoning feet begin to swell often up to over the knees; some may get even swollen arms, some even get a sudden very painful swelling of the face, sometimes it is accompanied by a fever. Do not be alarmed, because it is not dangerous, even if it is painful. The abscesses will soon dissolve if you crush the cranesbill (or any other geranium variety), and fix it to the painful areas. Drink diligently tea made from Lady's mantle (Alchemilla), or made from common Mallow (Malva Sylvesters), or the flowers and leaves of the Bindweeds (convolvus species). Instead of the cranesbill, you can make a poultice of a room geranium, crushed; it's the same plant and it will soon help.

JC: Sometimes we see this with folks who are new to hiking. They dive into a wilderness adventure without getting used to shorter hikes first. Cranesbill is a wild Geranium; it is astringent and tonic. Lady's Mantle is diuretic and astringent. Both of these will help reduce the swelling and fluid retention. Mallow shares those properties, but is more soothing in nature. It is very useful in helping the body cope with wounds, irritations and even serious infections. The Bindweed is also diuretic.

Simple remedy for calluses/corns

Many treat corns by cutting an onion into slices, soaking it in vinegar and putting a slice on the corns every night; helps many. In many cases one can blame vanity for developing corns as one wears shoes that are way too small.

JC: One could hardly enumerate all the virtues of the onion and the entire allium family. Warriors of old used to carry onions, leeks and garlic into battle – they provided food, kept digestion regular and were first aid for wounds. Fr. Künzle's advice on footwear is quite correct. Recently, one of the greatest of all baseball players, Chipper Jones of the Atlanta Braves, was forced to cut short his incredible career due to foot problems caused by his preference for wearing shoes a size too small. Good fitting shoes make for healthy feet, but it is even better to go barefoot as much as possible!

Treatment of children's illnesses

There are areas in Switzerland where, for decades, half of newborns usually die in their first year of life; and always in the same areas. It is not the climate to blame, but completely different circumstances; when circumstances are changed the mortality disappears as well. I know a pastor who investigated the cause of this mortality and soon he found out that the children lacked milk that God gave to the mothers; the pastor gathered the mothers, explained their duty, instructed them about the treatment of children diseases and was relieved to see the child mortality drop from 60 percent to 8 percent, this percentage has remained for years.

At first the pastor had his doubts whether it was appropriate for a clergyman to speak about health and illnesses; he therefore asked a doctor, a friend of his, to give a lecture, whereupon the latter, a person who has extensive knowledge, gave an excellent answer: "Why not you yourself? Did the Saviour only deal with purely spiritual things? Did he not heal every physical illness. Furthermore, you as a priest, have more authority than I over your people; if I speak, they would say, he only wants to earn money from us.

In response to this remark by the doctor, the priest reminded the mothers of their duty to give natural food to the children, and he instructed them how to treat children's diseases, what kind of food was appropriate, and how they should not keep children away from fresh air, water and light. Having this in mind, I will also briefly give you some advice.

1. Before giving birth. Many children are already ruined in the womb. Parents who have some addictions, such as alcoholism, or other severe disorders, etc. usually pass these traits on to their children. Mothers who enjoy dancing during pregnancy, or mothers who indulge in severe anger or are prone to great sadness or work too much, harm the child.

2. After giving birth. It is a requirement given from God that mothers breastfeed their children as long as possible; even indigenous peoples observe this custom. Mary, the virgin Mother of God most respected and admired by women, is especially praised for this reason in the Holy Scriptures. Unfortunately, there are now enough mothers who can no longer fulfill this sacred duty of nature because of weakness or illness or some fault of nature. I don't want to blame them. Much more numerous, however, are those mothers who, out of comfort, false shame and supercilious vanity, or arrogance, neglect this sacred duty or only fulfill it for a very short time, 8-14 days. They then use all kinds of artificial nutrition, but these cannot replace the milk of the mothers like a nanny cannot replace the mother.

Children who do not get the milk of their mothers usually develop intestinal catarrh, gouts and half of them die in the first year of their life.

JC: If only more modern women would follow Fr. Künzle's advice on this matter and stop following the advice of advertisers and drug companies, whose goal it is to create customers, not health! The maladies so common in America such as heart disease, diabetes, cancer and obesity, are not caused by a lack of nutritious food or poor living conditions. They are caused by the consumption of junk food and too many prescription drugs! It is a sad fact that children born just a few decades ago, even to mothers who smoked cigarettes and drank alcohol while pregnant (which one should absolutely not do) were often healthier and stronger than those born to modern women who spend fortunes on packaged, chemically laden food and eternities in doctors' offices, following the advice of "experts". Fr. Künzle is quite right in that God has given us all we need and the best foods in nature. I highly recommend the Weston A.

Price foundation, its cookbooks and papers on the subject of nutrition.

Children's illnesses

Preliminary remark. When children are ill with almost all children's diseases, especially rashes, eruptions, sores, measles, the children urinate too little. Every mother should pay attention to this first of all, because children will never say anything about it, not even a word. If too little urine comes out, it gets stuck in the body, forms lymph glands or acids or fever; yes, this can lead to severe eye and ear problems, or even to St. Vitus's dance and epilepsy. In the latter case, the excretory organs should be examined by a doctor.

It is very easy to cure too little urine in children. Give the child half a cup of Common couch roots (Triticum repens), once or twice a day and observe the following signs:

a) Rashes, eruptions, acids, abscesses, spots are due to inadequate quantities of dissolved water. External lubrication with ointments and bathing alone do not help. It means a child needs stronger diuretics. Common couch roots (triticum repens), alpine lady's-mantle (Alchymilla alpina), silver Mantle, Horsetail (Equisetum), Spiny Restharrow (ononis spinosa), should be given as teas separately or mixed, many times a day until the rashes disappear. For this I give lapidary to adults, the strongest blood cleansing herbal medication that exists.

b) In case of whooping cough, bathe the child twice a day in warm bath enriched with boiled pine twigs; rub the breast 7 to 12 times a day with our Filix (fern tincture); Every hour give him a sip of cough tea to drink (thyme, lemon balm, peppermint, common couch roots, sage).

c) A lot of children have worms. Against this, God created the small varieties of ferns that grow on the walls and on the rocks (Ruta murorum), the maidenhair fern (Capillus veneris). The large ferns are not suitable for children and even for adults they must be mixed with three times as many juniper berries. The children are given a cup of this tea in the morning on an empty stomach and should not eat anything for two hours; this is repeated for four to five days.

d) one can treat Diarrhea with blackberry leaves tea; they are green even in winter and can always be found at the edges of the forest; Edelweiss works even faster (four to five flowers, well boiled is enough quantity), the fastest remedy is the tea from tormentil (Potentilla erecta).

e) English disease. Children who at the age of one year are as weak like three month old ones, who at the age of two or more cannot stand are said to have the English disease. A very effective remedy, which helps in 90 percent of all cases, is to take pine twigs from the highest mountains, especially the twigs of the mountain pine (Pinus mugo), which spread along on the top rocks, simmer it for two to three hours and bathe the child in warm decoction for a quarter of an hour every day, for about four to eight weeks. The child is soon more lively, starts cooing, standing and jumping. Baths in the yellow willow rods or in the knotgrass (Polygonum aviculare) also help. Besides, give the child plenty of plantain syrup and common couch roots.

f) Preventive agents in the event of childhood diseases such as measles, scarlet fever, rubella, whooping cough. As soon as there is a threat to get infected, put two to three pieces of garlic or onions or Alpine leek in a bag and fix it on the child's neck; I know a family with 16 children who always used this prevention and were completely spared from all these children's illnesses; there is no superstition here at all, it is just the natural effect of these strong plants.

How kindly did Providence think of humanity when the plants were created!

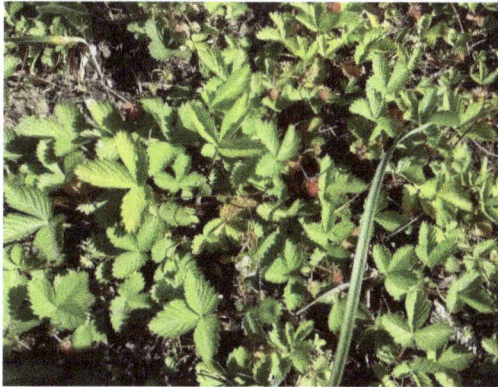

Wild Strawberry

g) Stomatitis and its remedies. There are many blisters in the mouth, sometimes with and sometimes without pus; this is often accompanied by severe toothache. Remedies: chew fresh rose petals and keep them in your mouth, or cranesbill, but do not swallow it, although it is not poison; or raspberry or blackberry shoots, boil these and rinse your mouth with this decoction; also chewing blueberry leaves or boiling them and rinsing the mouth will do the same; wild strawberry leaves and common Mallow (Malva sylvestris) can also be used. Thus there are enough simple and cheap remedies.

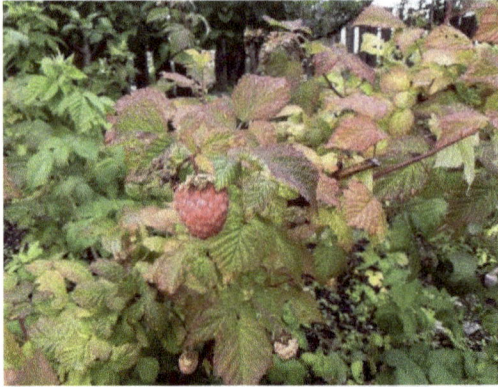

Raspberry

h) "Mummy, I have a stomach ache!" Who didn't whine like that as a child? That can be quickly cured. Boil caraway or anise in milk and give it to the child to drink; the winds will immediately find their way out and the "stomach ache" is gone.

i) Something is stuck in the child's throat, it cannot go either up or down. Put a finger or two down the child's throat and he will vomit anything that is in the way.

k) "A wasp has stung me!" Crushed mallow will instantly take away all the pain, even wet soil will help soon.

l) "Mummy, it hurts!" Wash the wound in fresh water, then take some plantain leaves, crush them, and put them on the wound; the wound will heal very quickly.

m) "Mummy, I have pinched myself!" "Pinching" is much worse than "Mummy hurts". The child should keep the finger as long as possible in ordinary oil or in olive oil; then use the white of the egg and wrap it round the finger.

n) Nail bed inflammation heals fastest when the child bathes the hand in herbal meadow hay water several times a day; in between you can apply any healing ointment.

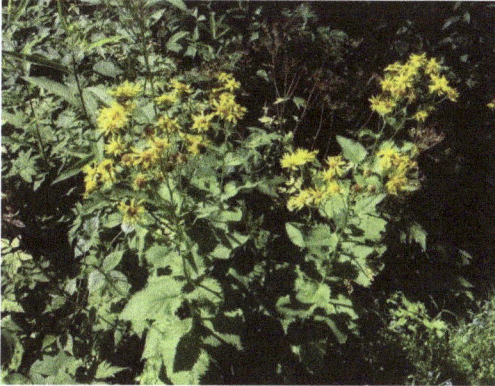

Alpine Ragwort

o) in case of diphtheria you have to call the doctor; until he arrives, wrap the child's neck with cold vinegar compresses. It is very important not to let the fever rise; as soon as it rises, wash the whole body with cold water. Then mix five tablespoons of Pimpinella root powder with twice as much honey, electuarium or syrup and give the child a full tablespoon every quarter of an hour. - Goldenrod (Solidago virga aurea) or the pagan magic herb wood ragwort (Senecio Fuchsii), is equally effective, both internally and externally; a Bavarian teacher healed over 5000 children with the latter remedy.

Use the same means against croup

p) Bed-wetting results from bladder weakness. The following mixture has proven to be effective: 1 part of St. John's wort, 1 part of yarrow, 3 parts of creeping tormentil (Potentilaa reptans) , 2 parts of knotgrass (polygonum aviculare), 1 part of juniper berries. The children are given a cup of that mixture twice a day.

Where strong sleep is assumed to be the cause, a handkerchief is tied around the child and the knot is tied in the middle of the back. When he is about to urinate, he turns over to his back and wakes up because of the knot. It has been proved to be true! Probatum est!

A lot of children's illnesses come from the fact that children sit on the damp soil and on stone stairs, even on the poisonous cement stairs that even cats avoid.

Above all, pray that dear Guardian Angels protect children every day and then they will be happy to protect them.

JC: The only things I would add to this is that tobacco is very effective against stings (chew a bit of natural tobacco up and apply it to the sting; the pain, itching and inflammation will quickly be reduced or go away entirely), and it is likely a good idea to keep a homeopathic remedy of Arnica on hand for use in all injuries and trauma. Arnica oil is also good, used externally only, for bruises and sprains.

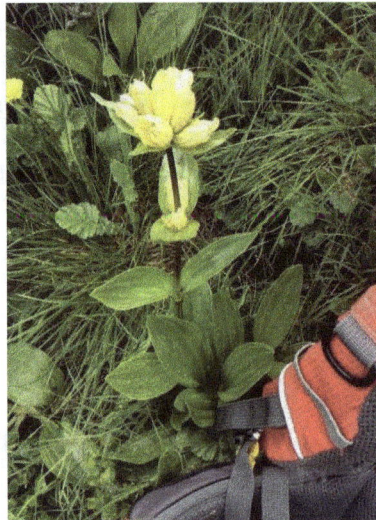

Gentian

Colic

requires immediate help, otherwise the person is lost. The patient feels terrible pain in the intestines, has no bowel movements and vomits everything.

Externally, soak a sheet, folded four times in hot water and place it on the abdomen.
Internally: a glass of real yellow gentian (Gentiana lutea) schnapps, but very warm; if you don't have this, boil milk with three cloves of garlic and five spoons of caraway. If even this does not help, the patient should drink a glass of St John's wort oil.

Caraway milk is another remedy for colic and for abdominal cold and even for an inflamed appendix. One squashes caraway, boils it well in milk, the milk is then well sifted and given warm to the patient every hour.

JC: Gentian is very stimulating to the digestive juices and organs. It is good to take a Gentian based bitters, daily, before each meal. This will help prevent such conditions and offers a wealth of other health benefits – increased appetite, preventing indigestion and bloating, it helps with allergies by helping the body digest proteins quickly so that an immune response is not triggered, is good for the liver and gallbladder, good to prevent diarrhea and constipation and good for blood sugar. Gentian has many other medicinal effects, as well. One should never be without bitters, whether the Swedish Bitters, a more simple Gentian bitters or even a few dandelion stems or bitter greens!

Recipe for people with lung diseases

God knows how many people suffer from lung diseases and coughing. Many even do not want to get well. They are too lazy to use a remedy for four weeks, the spoiled people despise everything that does not taste well. Of course, those cannot be helped.

Furthermore, if they are already weakened to such an extent that they are bedridden, no remedy would help any longer, no matter how much it is praised. However, there are still many, who still want to be cured and go out. For them I write down this tried out and tested recipe.

Finely chop green fir tree twigs or, if you can't get them, European spruce (picea abies) will also do and you chop it thinly. Fill 8-10 baskets and put them in the patient's bedroom or, if there is not enough space, hang them up like lamps; every evening before going to bed, stir and shake every basket so that the scent comes out.

If the twigs no longer smell after three to four weeks, replace them filled with the fresh ones.

I have seen tuberculosis patients who could only move with the help of sticks cured in this way.

In mountainous areas a much stronger and more effective variety of pines thrives, namely the dwarf mountain pine; it is hardly as tall as a man, but it spreads countless branches that crawl over the rocks up to the top of the tree line.

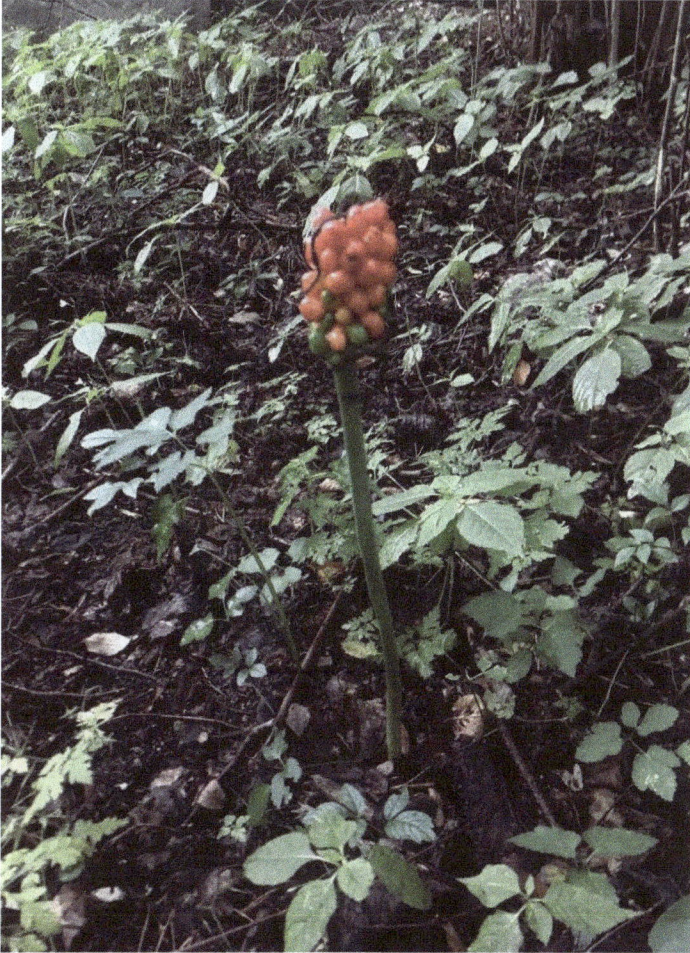

Arum

As internal medicine, I recommend the following syrup to all types
of lung patients, including those suffering from influenza:
3 handfuls of juniper green twigs,
3 handfuls of plantain,
1 handful of nettles,
1 handful of St. John's wort,
3 handfuls of Angelica,
1 handful of mullein,

1 handful of ground ivy
1 handful of peppermint,
1/2 handful of anise and fennel,
1 handful of Iceland moss
1 handful of speedwell,
2 handfuls of real lungwort
1/2 handful of arum leaves
1/2 handful of danewort roots
1/2 handful of burnet roots
Usage and treatment just like sirup for blood and stomach diseases.

We produce this with alpine varieties in the form of an extract under the name Angelika, which is pleasant to drink and has been proven to be a good remedy.

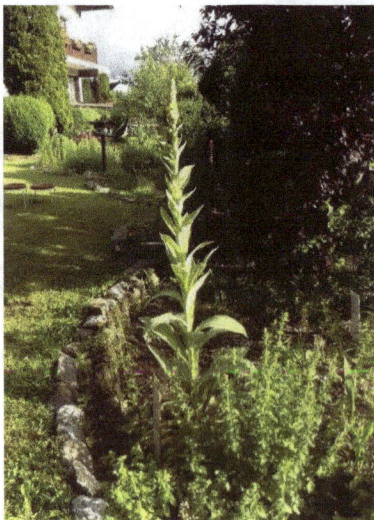

Mullein

JC: What an excellent protocol! It would take far too many words to extoll the virtues of each herb. But, suffice to say, Fr. Künzle has covered all the bases! Many of these herbs are both

tonic to the lungs and expectorant. All that is missing is pure mountain air!

Treatment of Tuberculosis

Uelis Sepp is 23 years old and has pulmonary consumption; he coughs on and on; in the evening he always has a little fever and coughs all night through; he can still walk around the house; he has already been to many doctors without success; they advise him to go to a sanatorium, but he just can't afford that. He wants to get well and would absolutely swallow anything if he thought it could help him.

1. Because Uelis Sepp can still walk around the house, nature is still helping him; as he wants to do everything that helps, one can help him. But if he were no longer able to walk outside the room or even if he was bedridden, all the effort would be in vain, as would be the case with pulmonary bleedings.

2. Uelis Sepp goes outside three times a day, into the healthy, dust-free air, if it is possible, he should stand under a fir tree, slowly and deeply breathes in with an open mouth and spreads out arms like on a cross so that the chest is expanded; as soon as his lungs are completely full, he folds both his hands as tightly as he can on his chest and breathes out; he repeats that ten to twelve times, always before taking a meal. This exercise ensures that the illness no longer destroys his lungs and so that those still healthy parts of the lungs remain intact.

3. Every hour Uelis Sepp takes a sip of the medicine made according to the recipe for lung patients. He can eat whatever he wants.

4. The kidneys and bladder of the lung patients usually work badly; as a result, entangled urine substances get into the lungs and new mucus is produced every day; no cure is possible before the kidneys and the bladder start working properly. The tea for lung patients drunk 2-3 weeks could help to make the kidneys and bladder function; Furthermore, warm herbs such as marjoram, thyme, mint and nettles are placed as a poultice as close as possible to the kidneys and to the bladder, and this bandage is worn for three to four weeks and during the cold season continuously. 10 - 20 warm hip baths in boiled pine or fir twigs strengthen the cure. This would make the kidneys and the bladder start working properly; more urine comes out; no more new mucus would develop in the lungs; the old mucus is excreted; without mucus, the Tuberculosis bacteria cannot multiply so quickly, the lungs become stronger and overcome the crisis. In case of a very advanced tuberculosis, however, there is no guarantee that this remedy will help.

JC: In the early 1900s, it was wrongly supposed that pine trees would offer the same tonic effect on the lungs as breathing in the scent of fir and spruce. For several years, I lived in the location of a former "Tuberculosis Retreat", in the piney sandhills region. There, I saw the worst and most widespread allergies and bronchial inflammations among the residents I have ever witnessed! Most people had swollen faces, red eyes and were constantly coughing and wheezing. The water was contaminated and even radioactive. Never have I seen an unhealthier population. Among the first books of Hippocrates was "On Airs, Waters and Places", which detailed how the environment of his world affect those who lived in it. We would all be very wise to choose to live in healthy environments, away from both pollution and natural irritants.

Runny nose and catarrh

Winter demonstrates its reign by gripping millions of people with the first cold. Strong and healthy people working outdoors usually manage to get rid of their catarrh quite soon. However, people who stay inside, in workshops, factories, etc., are far more severely affected; if they are of poor health, the catarrh will not disappear and turns into hoarseness and congestion in the lungs. Thank God the Creator, who has placed numerous healing powers in plants for these ailments too.

If you have a cold and catarrh, in the evening before you go to bed drink a good portion of well-boiled tea made from plantain, cowslip, Lady's Mantle and peppermint. If you do this at the very beginning when you start feeling the symptoms, you will be healthy the following morning; if, on the other hand, you have missed the moment, drink this tea more often throughout the day (always warm), then usually you should be free of catarrh by the evening.

When the cold sets in, people have to dress differently; all animals are provided by the good Lord either with warmer clothing, such as rabbits, foxes, weasels, chickens, ducks, etc., or are sent to warmer places, such as migratory birds, or are hidden in cracks, holes, caves and sheltered places, such as marmots and lots of insects. That is a hint for people; here it means keeping feet warm and dry, head and neck free. Just no neckerchiefs or thick scarves around the neck, because these make the neck less resistant and turns it into a safe breeding place for all kinds of neck ailments. People who have got used to cold water throughout the summer (they wash the whole body in cold water!) and sleep with the window open are less prone to changes in the weather than water-shy people and they are less sensitive than those who lack fresh air.

Children who have run around barefoot during the summer can stand cold three times as much and are three times more resistant to cold than the spoiled and pampered children who wear shoes and stockings as symbols of nobility even in midsummer. If they are still freezing at 40 degrees Celsius and need stockings, for heaven's sake, which bearskin will be thick enough at minus 10 degrees! But these doll children always look pale like sacks of flour, light as feathers and frail like coffee cups; hardly released from school, they often have to go to doctors, wear scarfs and are packed in blankets in winter like hooded poachers, they develop anemia and headaches and have eternal toothaches; when such dolls enter into wedlock, just like a fly falls into hot water, then the man has enough music throughout his life, because he has a lamenting organ in the house, and a new voice is added with each birth.

JC: I was first introduced to the German Folk Medicine practices of walking barefoot in the dew and even snow, bathing in cold water and sleeping with the windows open to breathe fresh, clean, cool air, by an old man I met on a trail. He was tall and strong, though elderly. His pace of hiking was faster than mine, although I was in my teens, and he talked constantly without lacking breath. He came from an immigrant family, who practiced Fr. Kneipp's protocols. He was strong and fit, mentally sharp and had never had a serious cold or flu in his entire life! Do not take this advice on "strengthening the constitution" too lightly!

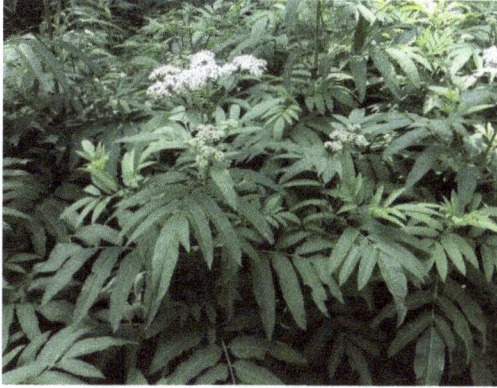

Valerian

Toothache

Once the teeth have started to produce pus, so-called puss teeth, herbs are no longer of any help; the faster you pull them out the better.

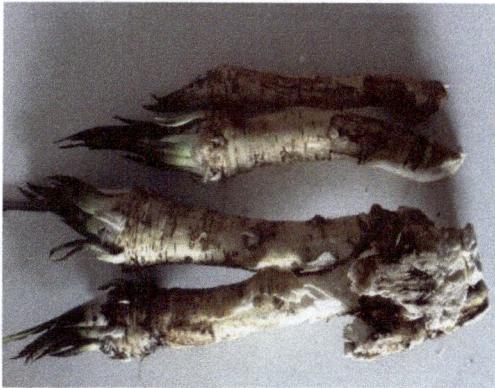

Horseradish

Pain relievers:
1. All types of plantain (Broadleaf, Ribwort, Hoary), boiled and gargle the mouth with it, it relieves the pain.
2. Lady's Mantle or Alpine Mantle provide a quick help when

boiled and gargled.

3. Horseradish, grated and put on linen and applied externally, helps almost immediately.

4. All kinds of peppermints, boiled and gargled, have the same effect.

5. Tormentil or creeping cinquefoil, boiled and gargled.

6. Common houseleek, chewed and kept in the mouth, relieves the pain instantly.

7. Also Meadowsweet, both leaves and blossoms, cooked and gargled, helps.

8. Valerian root, boiled and gargled (but do not swallow too much!) also helps.

I consider fern tincture to be the most effective remedy for toothache; it works instantly; we produce it under the legally protected name Filix.

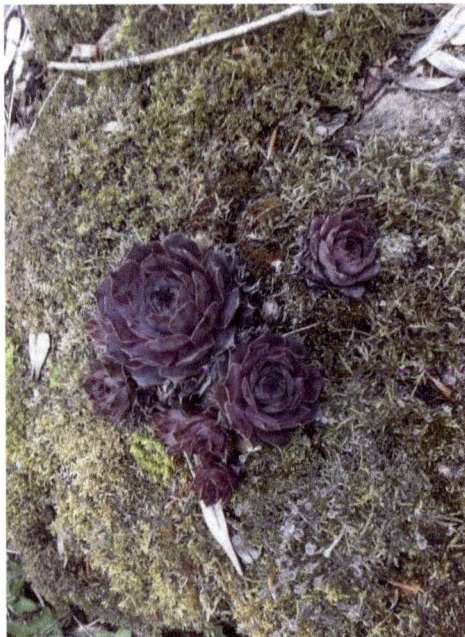

Houseleek

My advice. Take one or more of these herbs, crush them, put them in schnapps, expose it to the sun, strain it after ten days and store the liquid in bottles. When you have a toothache, mix one spoonful with five spoonfuls of water and gargle your mouth with it, this will help you.
How many simple and inexpensive means has God provided for a suffering that affects almost everyone!

Prevention. Wash your face every morning with pure cold water, dry it only after five minutes; this calms people down who otherwise cannot find any remedy any longer.

JC: Clove is also good for toothache, but it can be a bit irritating. Yarrow roots, "pickled" in vodka are said to be most effective.

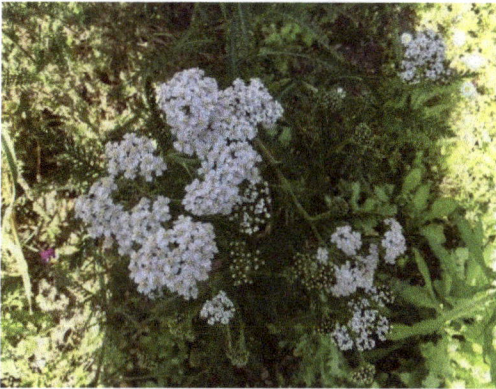

Yarrow

Hemostasis in slight and severe injuries

At first, sudden injuries with severe blood loss cause great confusion. If there is no doctor nearby, you usually don't know how to stop the severe bleeding. May everyone remember the following simple but safe procedure: Take a wad of cotton wool, dip it in hot, naturally pure water and place it on the wound. The success is surprising; even if the artery is injured, the bleeding stops immediately. If you apply a cotton wad alone or if you dip it in cold water, you will not have the same effect (Find a surgeon).

JC: To this, I would add a few remedies to stop bleeding. Perhaps the most effective and rapid is powdered Cayenne Pepper. This is excellent first aid, as it stops bleeding, causing coagulation and also treats shock. Tincture of yarrow and a homeopathic remedy of Arnica are also good to have on hand. The spores of the puffball mushroom act somewhat like Cayenne. Pine pitch is an excellent remedy, helping to stop the bleeding and disinfect the wound.

Blood and stomach diseases

In case of such diseases the right herbs work much better than all kinds of artificial medicine. Stomach and blood are so related to each other just like both eyes. When the stomach does not digest properly, the liver and kidneys cannot excrete properly and the illness begins; thus the intestines also suffer, and consequently many substances, not properly processed, get into the blood.

Centaury works best for reflux.

Fennel, caraway, anise, sprinkled onto the food ease belching, bloating and fullness problems.
For persistent diarrhea yarrow, mallow, shepherd's purse, Lady's mantle, leaves of blackberries, raspberries and blueberries help when used for a longer period of time.

Plantain and juniper help best to cure skin problems like abscesses, eruptions, eczema.

A good syrup for blood and stomach problems:

3 handfuls of green juniper twigs, 5 handfuls of plantain, 2 handfuls of nettles, 2 handfuls of St. John's wort, 1 handful of yarrow, 1 handful of peppermint, 1/2 handful of caraway, 1/2 handful of centaury, 1 handful of dead nettles (white, red, yellow), 1/2 handful of Masterwort root.

With the exception of dead nettles, boil all the herbs for two hours; the last quarter of an hour add dead nettles; strain the herbs after two hours, add to the liquid a good amount of white sugar and let everything simmer for another hour. Then let it cool down, pour it into bottles and jars, seal well and keep in a cool place.

How much water is to be added? As much as the herbs can absorb.

How to use it? Half a cup every morning on an empty stomach and half a cup every night before going to bed. Even better if you take a tablespoon every hour, for four weeks.

It is unbelievable how this remedy helps weak people, dying people or people who feel low, to regain strength and health.

The author has put together this recipe after much experimenting. However, he uses only alpine varieties of herbs, as these are much stronger, he boils the syrup for up to 24 hours and thus produces an extract that can be diluted five to ten times. It is sold under the name "Johannistropfen".

JC: Again, I also recommend taking digestive bitters before meals. These herbs are excellent for all the complaints lists, but with bitters and some regular naturally fermented foods, most of those complaints will never arise! Natural, "lacto-fermented" sauerkraut and pickles, water kefir, milk kefir, kombucha,

unpasteurized yogurt, kvass, etc will do more for digestion and immunity than most other remedies combined. The more we learn about our "gut micro-biome", all those bacteria and fungi, the more we realize just how essential they are for health. Antibiotics and environmental toxins disrupt, what is essentially, the heart of our natural immunity. The lack of healthy gut flora leads to sickness, disease, inflammation and even cognitive decline. As one doctor who respects natural health put it, "the more closely we look at the human body, the less of us there actually is... probiotic bacteria and fungi partner with our own cells to keep us healthy. One can see this happening before our eyes, when we make ferments – as the probiotic culture establishes itself in whatever is being ferments, from wine to pickles, it will outcompete and even fight off other types of bacteria that would contaminate and spoil the ferment. The probiotics literally colonize the medium and fight off the invaders so long as they are healthy. Make keeping them healthy a top priority!

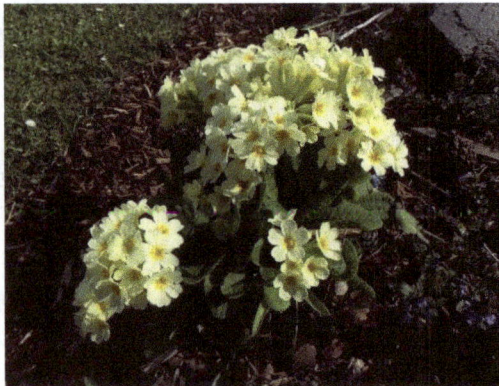

Cowslip

Mixtura professoralis. - Professor's tea (name protected by law)

This is the name I have given to the tea, which is mainly intended for people who, like professors, commanders, captains, preachers, catechists, teachers, porters at train stations, town criers, etc., have to speak a lot and loudly and therefore need a safe, fast-acting means to prevent or cure a runny nose, catarrh, hoarseness, toothache, headache; it also reduces the tendency to develop facial erysipelas and swelling of the tonsils.

It is a very pleasant and tasty tea that surpasses Chinese tea in terms of taste and is completely harmless to the nerves in the sense that it does not activate like the Chinese tea, but it soothes, so that it can be served as a family tea to everyone.

It is composed of the following alpine herbs:
1. Primula officinalis, fragrant cowslip,
2. Alchymilla alpina, Alpine Lady's mantle
3. Dryas octopetala, Mountain avens
4. Geum reptans, creeping avens,
5. Potentilla aurea, dwarf yellow cinquefoil
6. Meum mutellina, Alpine lovage
7. Plantago Alpina, Alpine plantain,
8. Mentha piperita, peppermint,
9. Triticum repens, coach grass root

The herbs indicated with 2, 3, 4, 5 belong to the Potentilaceae family and are somewhat radioactive; this is where their healing power probably comes from.

You boil the tea for half an hour, add sugar according to your taste and drink it warm as much as you want. Before you get used to it, it is better to take it during lunch time rather than before going to bed, because at the beginning it causes excessive urination which washes out the catarrhal substances.

This tea is not easy to collect and it is expensive, as many plants such as the Alpine lovage, the Alpine Plantain, the creeping avens, can only be found very high up in the Alps, but you can buy them in the herb depot in Zizers (Switzerland).

This tea removes the strongest cold within a few hours. People with cavities in their teeth, suffering from toothache every time the weather changes, are relieved by regular enjoyment of this tea. The same tea also cures diarrhea, bladder and urinary ailments and is therefore very beneficial for older people. Because of the herbs 2, 3, 4, 7 it is highly recommended after falls, bumps and internal injuries; however, in this case one must drink 1 to 2 liters per day.
This tea is also recommended to all women after childbirth because it prevents fever, inner heat, inflammation and strengthens the muscles. Herbs 2,3,4 are particularly helpful.

JC: This tea is very astringent and anti-inflammatory; it is an excellent cold and allergy remedy.

Heart troubles.

Pain in the heart and anxiety quite often result from hard stool; in these eternal meat-eating times this problem is a terribly frequent one. The fig cure helps here.

If there is no constipation, but if you were previously suffering from foot cramps and now no longer, then the ailment is of spasmodic origin; footbaths in fern root decoction could help.

If neither is the case, did you exhaust yourself too much, did you run a race with an express train, or did you run down from the mountain top as if ten Cossacks were chasing you? Then, you are allowed to believe that you have heart problems. In this case you have to slow down your life for a while, sleep a little longer, don't run, don't fuss, don't lift heavy items, avoid alcoholic beverages like poison, and wash the area around the heart once or twice a day with water and vinegar.

In case of heart-attacks, you should immediately apply cold water and vinegar compresses to the area around the heart.

The following recipe is effective for a weak heart, for an oedema and for calcification of the heart: 5 parts chickweed (Cerastium or Stellaria varieties) 5 parts Creeping avens, 2 parts alpine Lady's mantle, 1/2 part wormwood; drink half a cup five times a day. Just ask for Pastor Künzle's heart tea.

JC: Fr. Künzle's advice on bathing the chest with water and vinegar may seem odd, but it is based in the fact that with inflammation comes heat. An injured, enlarged or weakened heart generally does show signs of inflammation. Many people who followed Fr. Kneipp's advice of cold water treatments for heart ailments swear by their effectiveness. For the skeptic, I can only say, "It is worth a try", as such a treatment could do no harm. As for his advice on sleep though, that is essential. Most people simply do not get enough sleep. As a result, their hearts are stressed, their brains are tired, their liver does not get the opportunity to do its night-time job of cleaning the blood, and as such, the blood becomes acidic. This leads to more inflammation, poor mineral absorption, blood sugar issues, hormone imbalance, auto-immune disorders and yes, heart disease. Too often, such exhausted people turn to caffeine and sugar to keep them going. This compounds the problem. In fact, the only cure they may need is sleep. Many chronic conditions

have been cured by simply going to bed earlier and (if possible) sleeping a bit later. Fr. Kneipp would insist one sleep with the windows open for fresh air, and I am sure he was correct in that advice. The average person needs eight and a half hours of sleep for the liver to do its work, and many need even more.

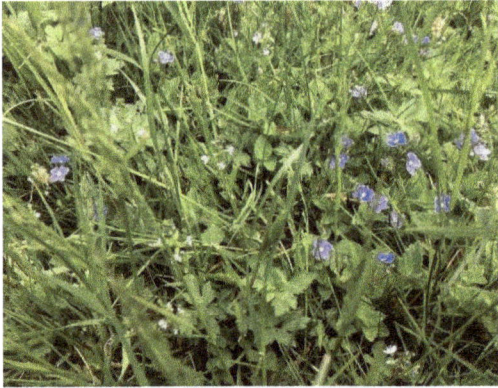

Heath Speedwell

Headache

often comes from an upset stomach; people having headaches often suffer from hard stools and regurgitation after eating. The gases which normally come out with a normal bowel movement cannot be set free because of the hard stool and then rise to the head. A regular fig cure could help.

Others have a spasmodic headache, which can be recognized by the fact that these people used to suffer a lot from foot and calve cramps, by the time they have headaches, cramps in the feet and calves have already disappeared quite some time ago. In this case, foot baths with the fern roots could help, for sure.

Finally a headache can result from a temporary exertion, also from catarrh, unhealed facial erysipelas, from the teeth, from swellings on the head. This is where the "professor's tea" would help.

People who usually work late into the night, students, scholars, railway officials, people in eternal "hustle and bustle", who do not have enough sleep and live like this for months, in the end develop an anxiety headache. Speedwell (Veronica officinalis), even more so Veronica fruticulosa is sometimes quite good for this ailment; by the way, one can say, enough, get away from all intellectual activities, away from the noise, away from the office and away from the city into the country, as high into the mountains as possible, lots and lots of exercise in the fresh air, and do that until you can sleep peacefully again. Quiet climatic health resorts, where there aren't many people, no pianos and no dogs, but lots of fir trees and murmuring brooks; only that can still help.

JC: In Fr. Künzle's time, one did not have the leading cause of headache we "advanced" modern folks have, computers. Whether from eye strain, or the spectrum of light emitted from screens, or even stressful communications, there is no doubt that a computer can and does cause many headaches. Turn it off. Turn off your phone. Turn off the television. Make time in your day to garden or go fishing. Actually, talk with friends or family, face to face, during meals. Take an after dinner walk. Read for 30 minutes before bed or do something else to naturally "unwind". Beyond that though, many food additives can cause headaches. MSG can wreak havoc on the brain for many people and, is often hidden under deceptive names. Processed and preserved foods are made for shelf life and often contain aldehydes and rancid fats. Diet, sleep and moderate exercise can go a long way in preventing many headaches.

Beware of cement floors!

It is now fashionable to lay cement floors in kitchens, hallways, basements, laundry rooms, butcher shops, etc. For 90 percent of the people who have to stand and walk there, these cement floors are the cause of continuous ailments in the throat, teeth, head, swallowing, a cause of tremendous cramps, rheumatism, lumbago, sciatica. Women who have to sweep such floors and who kneel on them without a board often develop terrible pains. Late arrivals in overcrowded churches who have to stand on bare cement floor for the entire duration of the service, often with their shoes still wet, then complain of all kinds of pains on the following day. Anyone who has to work on cement floors should immediately lay a thick board or cork linoleum over it. If you cannot do that, put on shoes with wooden soles. From October to May you should only mop such floors, never sweep them or you ask the employer to cover the costs of medical expenses and compensation for pains and suffering in advance. The Health commissions should look into this!
If you can afford it, you should immediately have a wooden floor or thick cork linoleum laid. Even pigs, dogs and cats get ill on such floors. So beware of the cement floors! Never let children sit on them, it will always result in a cough and fever.

JC: Of such hard floors being the cause of, "cramps, rheumatism, lumbago, sciatica" I can certainly attest! I worked on such floors for many years prior to becoming self employed. Back then, even wearing good shoes with cushioned insoles, my legs and back were exhausted and I was in agony after only 8 hours. Now, an 8 hour day is a short work day – those who work for themselves often work much longer hours. But, I rarely experience the type of pain and tiredness I did when I was younger. Even hard wood floors and stony ground have some natural give to them. I wish more employers and builders would

realize that they may have healthier, happier, harder working employees simply by installing different flooring.

Chocolate and cocoa

is loved by all children, whether small or big, whenever they are given a few cents, they would buy chocolate, and if money is stolen from their parents, it will certainly be spent on chocolate and cookies. In factories and in female shops, many people eat these black cookies all day long like old horses; you will find chocolate papers and chocolate pictures appearing as signs of this eating culture everywhere in the streets. Once every Liseli and Babeli (female names) gets the right to vote and if you want to become a member of Parliament, buy them a cartload of chocolate and they will enthusiastically support you, no matter whether you are a red socialist or even blacker than an old Jesuit.

"Herbalist, what do you think of the chocolate"? a mother asked me. Here is my opinion based on experience:

1. Chocolate is useful for those who suffer from diarrhea because it blocks diarrhea
2. It is very useful for Chocolate = manufacturers who multiply like horse flies in the summer.
3. It is of particular benefit to doctors, who thereby get a large number of customers. Chocolate causes constipation, eating chocolate regularly causes permanent constipation; constipation, however, is the mother of half of all illnesses. Chocolate children sooner or later will all develop stomach problems. So now you know what to think of the chocolate treat. Whoever wants to spoil the health of the children, just give them chocolate often; if you want to do them good, give them all kinds of fruits, nuts, figs, oranges, dates, apples, pears, etc.

JC: We can only hope that our federal "elected representatives" never learn of this…. if they begin buying votes and trading favors, we are in BIG trouble! (stated sarcastically)

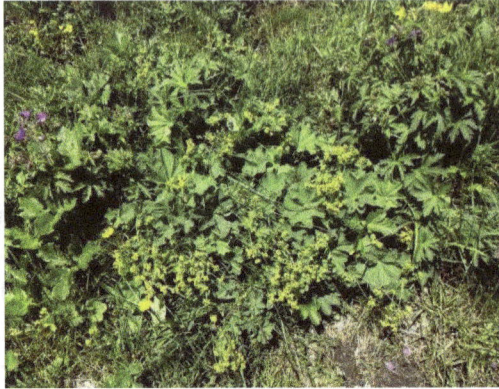

Lady's Mantle

Edema

is curable at the beginning. The patient is given urination stimulating herbs: horsetail and Lady's mantle. If one has no fever, one can be given tea from butterbur powdered roots; the larger and thicker is the leaf, the more effective is the root. People who tend to have edema should drink horsetail (of any kind) and Lady's mantle tea at least once a week.

Birch Leaves

Continued consumption of birch leaves (Betula alba), boiled with wine, drunk in the morning and evening, also helps against edema. Others find the blossoms of the Meadowsweet boiled in wine even better. In addition, the roots of the Restharrow (Ononis spinosa), wall hawkweed (Hieracium murorum) and Alpine hawkweed (hieracium alpinum), and especially the corn silk, have an excellent effect. You can get a mixture of all these herbs by the name "Pastor Künzles edema tea".

JC: Edema is, essentially, fluid retention. The most sure sign of it is when the lower extremities, such as the ankles, are puffy and swollen... and, if you press into them with a finger, it leaves an indentation that is slow to fill back in. If not treated quickly, much tissue damage can occur. Diuretic and astringent herbs can be of help.

Sweaty feet

is the healthiest of all the diseases. These people get rid of all illnesses through the soles of their feet. One should therefore never get rid of it directly, otherwise serious and incurable diseases will develop and stay until the sweat is restored. The latter can be achieved with difficulty through the help of feet bath in herb hay. Sweaty feet should only be gently reduced, but never, never, never by taking cold feet baths, but by cleansing the kidneys by drinking diuretic herbs, such as silver Lady's mantle, horsetail, corn silk, coach grass, etc.

JC: The skin is an often-overlooked excretory organ. Skin is our largest organ, and much like the kidneys in function. We sweat out toxins, waste and sickness. One reason why illness is more frequent in winter is that we not only sweat less, but our skin is more heavily covered and has less chance to "breathe". Fr. Kneipp's Water Treatments can be very helpful during such times. Oddly enough, a 5 – 10 minute foot bath in ice cold tater, especially if white vinegar is added to the water, followed by putting on warm socks and covering the feet with a blanket, can cause the feet to sweat profusely. Other times, sweating may be induced with diaphoretic herbs, a hot, deep bath into which fresh, sliced/crushed ginger has been added or, of course, a hot sauna especially with some juniper, can be a great relief. Such sweats leave one feeling relaxed, healthy, usually a little sleepy, but with a feeling of lightness and relief.

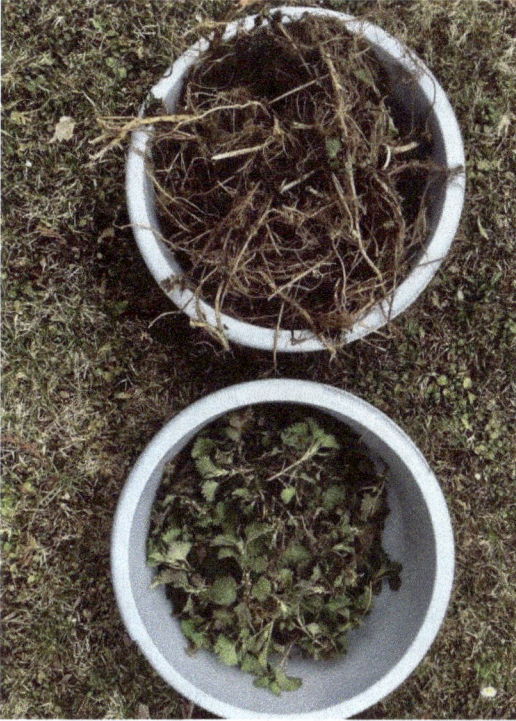

Nettle Root

For gallstones

take nettle roots and also leaves; boil them in milk for a while and drink it. It removes the gallstones and also drains away water; also dandelion roots help for sure, too. Ivy leaves have an even stronger effect when boiled in wine (not in water!); take a tablespoonful of this decoction after each meal, but no more, otherwise it has a bad effect on the stomach.

JC: Often, appearance conscious women suffer most from gallstones. The reason is diet. When one wishes to lose weight, the easiest meal to skip is breakfast. This, is especially true with the modern, rushed schedule. Perhaps a cup of coffee is all one has, or something sweet. The gallbladder is stimulated by sour

and bitter flavors, along with the consumption of fats. Simply having one's salad for breakfast, with bitter greens and an olive oil vinaigrette, could go a long way in preventing such a painful condition, while stimulating the metabolism and enhancing weight loss. Often, if I awake with no appetite... my nature being more in accord with a big, sausage egg and bacon laden "brunch", I have my Swedish bitters along with a dill pickle and spoonful of olive or sesame oil. This odd combination feels great on the stomach and along with a cup of plain kombucha, really gets the system going. Then, I can sip on my coffee for an hour or two before I really get hungry.

Chilblains

and cracked hands are healed safely and quickly through mistletoe baths or compresses; the herb should be thoroughly boiled. We also have a well-proven ointment available under the name "Frigor" (protected by law).

JC: Again, I must warn against using American Mistletoe. Aside from being very poisonous, the American Mistletoe generally has the opposite effects of European Mistletoe. The European Mistletoe is calming, pain reducing, etc. The American Mistletoe causes extreme, painful muscle cramping and spikes in blood pressure that can cause stroke. Ginger, Rosemary and Cayenne Pepper are more accessible herbs for Americans to use for chilblains.

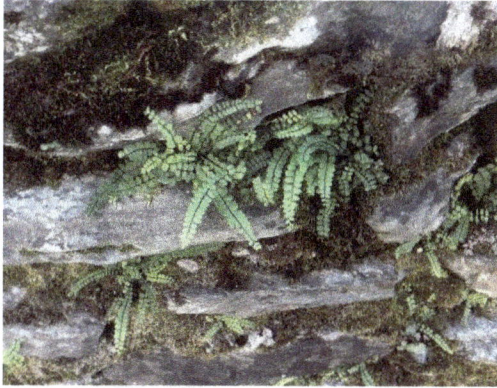

Rapid healing of rheumatoid arthritis, (rheumatism, sciatica, lumbago).

Suddenly you can no longer walk; or you can no longer lift your arm; this "Plague" drills and gnaws in the shoulder blade and in the joints; no plaster, no ant spirit, no juniper spirit can help. The doctor thinks you should stay in bed for three to four weeks; meanwhile he wants to treat you with Salicylic acid. But you have had this Salicylic acid two years ago.

It healed your rheumatism, but it damaged your stomach.

If you want to get rid of the evil "guest" quickly, at the longest in five to seven days, do it like this:

1. Take one or two fern roots, which are still fresh, also on the inside (dried and cut ones lose their strength within a few days), cut them up into small pieces, but do not wash them, put everything in a sack and put it or tie this sack on to the painful area and leave it there until the pain is gone. Quite often all the pain is gone after just half a day. - If the whole back is affected, you need more roots and a longer sack and you have to lie on it.

2. If you cannot or do not want to stay in bed, then bathe and massage the sick limb for half an hour in the fern root bath on the same day (but not on the same half day).

3. When in bed apply the juniper compress, over the painful areas.

4. Before going to sleep, either drink good mulled wine or elderberry tea or best would be to drink Meadowsweet (Spiraea ulmaria), boiled in wine.

Do that for four to six days and you will be cured. But if your rheumatism has not appeared all of a sudden, but has already been there for years, or if you are 60 or more years old yourself, take the full herbal bath on one day, take the juniper on the next day, drink daily tea from birch leaves, Meadowsweet, Spiny restharrow and Lady's bedstraw, take a sip about every hour, then you can be cured in three to six weeks, depending on the depth and length of your illness. I have seen 70-year-old people suffering and distorted from gout got cured after having undergone this treatment in the spa building "Wangs" near Sargans (Switzerland). Many are cured also without baths only by drinking rheumatoid tea and by rubbing fern ointment (Filix) daily on the kidneys and bladder area several times every day.

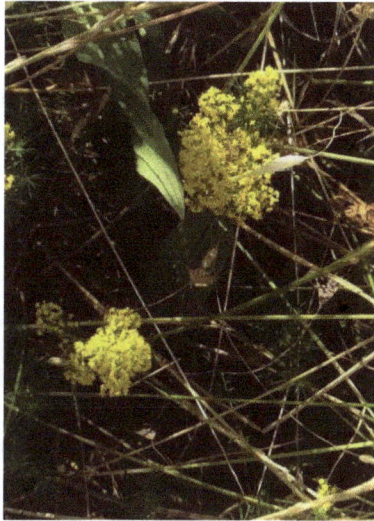
Lady's Bedstraw

JC: Once again, Fr. Künzle recommends Fern... it is a wonder that ferns are not more used in modern herbalism. Maude Grieve listed several in her A Modern Herbal, that became very influential in Britain and America following the World Wars. One remedy that I doubt Fr. Künzle knew about though, is quite effective. Natural tobacco added to a bath or to soak the inflamed area is very good to reduce pain and inflammation. However, one absorbs nicotine through the skin, so it should not be used by people who have overcome an addiction to tobacco or for very long, as too much nicotine can make you nauseous and dizzy. In small amounts, tobacco is excellent for painful stings such as from wasps or hornets, and for painful joints and muscles.

Nervousness!

Nervousness is never a cause but an effect, therefore this misery must be treated differently. The cause of nervousness is a disease substance that wraps and penetrates the nerves and thus makes them sick. This disease substance almost always arises from poor activity of the kidneys, the bladder, and more often of the stomach and intestines and the liver. If one wants to cure nervousness, then one should do the following:

1. First of all one should repair the diseased organs with the help of the herbs described above;

2. The disease substance must be extracted, which is best done with the help of a Milanese plasters (Muches de Milan), which you can also get from us. These are placed two on either side of the ears if the reason of nervousness is in the head; if the nerves of the back are also effected, three plasters are placed on each side of the back, within a period of 12-18 hours the plasters will suck out lots of inflammation liquid from the affected areas; if you stick a needle into them, up to one Liter of liquid can come out. If the plaster does not pull out the liquid, then the blood circulation is poor and must be restored by consuming Lapidar for four weeks, then the plaster works well.

Nervousness is most common in mentally stressed people who don't have enough sleep. If the body is not cleaned by the kidneys, the disease substance which they should extract finds its way into the head.

There are also nervous people who neither are involved in mental activity nor are deprived of enough sleeping time. These have either problems in their stomach or intestines or kidneys. Then these organs have to be treated.

JC: Again, Fr. Künzle's advice is centered on good digestion, excretion and plenty of sleep. We take such things for granted

too often and at our peril.

Meat, meat, meat!

Meat for lunch, meat in the evening, a sausage during the break; meat, no matter how expensive it is; Meat, even if the butcher can hardly find it! Meat even for the kids! Meat until the parliaments are at a loss and no longer know where to get the meat from! Alas, the stomach can no longer work, the intestines are weakened, constant constipation or terrible diarrhea; you run to the doctors, to the pharmacists, to all quacks and speculators on this side or beyond the great water, swallow pills, take poisons, have massages, bathes, moan and groan, but you still shout: "I want meat, meat, meat every day!"

It is considered to be posh, to have at least three different kinds of meat on the table, each time on a different plate, of course, but unfortunately not in a different stomach; The "bourgeois cuisine" demands two kinds of meat. Only one kind of meat is considered to be a sign of poverty or uncivilized.

But the head is blocked, the body so full, the sleep so restless, the mood so bad. Therefore one needs a strong wine, or a schnapps, that splits everything! But the constipation won't go away. So back to the doctor! But again meat, meat, meat! Meat under all circumstances!

Until a hundred years ago, the Catholic Church was able to keep to two days of fasting every week on Friday and on Saturday, on which all meat consumption was forbidden; in addition, there was the compulsory fasting, three days each quarter of a year; from Ash Wednesday to Easter the abstinence from meat was required for forty days, with the exception of Sundays. There was a time when these fasts were kept throughout Christendom; in those days little or nothing was known about constipation nor was the long row of the diseases known, which constipation causes; the meat was cheaper, life lasted longer and the physical appearance was better.

In the 19th century, however, pastors and chaplains by the hundreds and thousands persuaded the Pope to soften the prohibition of meat by shouting: "The prohibition can no longer be followed, everybody wants meat, we are being stoned, for God's sake, we have to make the requirements milder!" And then dispensation was given, so that now only every Friday is left; of the forty days of fasting, however, only the last three days of Holy Week remained. And how hard it is to keep to that! How many don't even do without meat on Friday!

God's commandments and the Church are founded on nature. The law of Nature and positive law ultimately come from the same lawmaker, the creator of nature, and breaking the commandments is followed by revenge. Those who stand on their head, have blood in their heads, even if they have forced exemptions from the requirements to be granted, and whoever cuts himself will bleed, even if he has the exemption paper in his pocket, and whoever does not follow healthy food habits, which find their reason in human nature, will have to cope with the damages to his body.

But then I can hear moaning from all sides: "I can hardly endure the foods from Lent in particular; they are heavy on my stomach, cause acid belching, make me feel sick, so meat, meat!"

What foods do you eat for Lent, you sighing brothers? Well, eggs, pastries, cheese, everything dripping with butter or margarine or some other fat. Yes, if you chop wood after such a meal or dig up the field or bring in hay, you will be able to digest it, if your stomach has not already been weakened by the eternal meat eating.

However, if your work does not involve a lot of physical effort, you have to avoid the above-mentioned heavy meals. Shall I suggest you to take light and tolerable and yet nutritious fasting foods, this is what I together with Pastor Kneipp advise:

Habermus, grain mash (Brenntar or Schwarzer Brei), the food of our fathers. "Come on, children, eat grain mash, grow and increase your weight," this is what Hebel, the Alemannic poet, proclaims. I don't like modern poets, pianos and school laws, these products of an overstimulated culture, but Hebel is not a modern moonlight poet praising hollow trees and waitresses! Lord, grain mash, Habermus! I don't like that! Why not? It tastes bad. But does the headache, the burning stomach, the belching and an early death taste good? Do pills and bottles taste good? Try it for eight days, then you'll get used to it and then you will get used to and prefer your grain mash to all highly praised dishes and sweets.

People who are used to grain mash, are healthy like Bulgarians, have a sense of humor like a shepherd kid, sleep like a bear, but they are neither like pungent bites nor pricking. Children who eat grain mash are red-cheeked, chubby and look at you like God's dear sun looks at hay.

2. Barley, peas and beans boiled together, a little celery, parsley, chives in it, make a tasty strong soup; two to three full bowls eaten at lunchtime fill the strongest man and keep him healthy. This is the soup of our fathers from the natural ancient times; this soup turns men into iron - and women even after their twelfth child are still as strong and as healthy as oaks.

3. All kinds of vegetables, fresh and dried fruit, dried apples and pears, dry plums, figs, and grapes make an easily digestible and good fasting dish. And even more potatoes, fresh from the pan! Meat should not be eaten as a rule but as an exception, as it was the case in times gone by. Only in such a way constipation with all the ensuing pains can be safely and permanently healed or prevented.

4. All the Maggi products in which vegetables of all kinds are produced in an easily digestible way are very beneficial.

5. Those who have it and can afford it, will cherish milk soups, roasted flour soup, etc. as high quality fasten soups.

I knew a man in his forties who was constipated like an old bottle of wine; no pill and no poison helped him anymore. Business took him to northern France where he had to stay for a quarter of a year and live among the farmers. There he no longer got meat, but milk, lots of vegetables, grain mash (Habermus), thin beer. This way of life restored him completely.

If we strictly kept to the forty-day fasts and ate fasting foods of our fathers, 60 percent of all medicines would be superfluous. Our forefathers on certain days had the "Magro stretto": during these days nothing made from warm-blooded animals was allowed to be eaten, neither eggs, nor butter, nor milk and cheese, thus only entirely vegetarian food. That cured even the most constipated sinners.

So here again Pastor Kneipp's principle: "Back to nature!"

JC: This dietary philosophy is very much in keeping with the tradition of Monastic medicine. From Saint Hildegard to Frs. Kneipp and Fr. Künzle, we find strong advice toward grains,

vegetables and fish. There is no doubt that both moderation in eating and eating a large variety of seasonal foods provides one with good nutrition and good digestion. Fasting was also very much a part of their lives, and we are once again realizing the benefits of "periodic fasting" today... in fact, it has become quite trendy. It should be stressed though, that none of these Catholic healers promoted a vegetarian or vegan diet. "All things in moderation." Fr. Künzle was quite right in predicting the eventually relaxation of the Catholic rule of abstaining from meat on Fridays. Unfortunately, obtaining fresh fish and seafood was not possible for many people as populations moved inland and away from historic port cities. It is also the case, that the fish that was once the humble food of the common man, became far too expensive for many (especially large Catholic) families. For better or worse, the rule was laxed. Catholics are still called to fast on Ash Wednesday and Good Friday, only eating one evening meal which may include fish but not meat. Two snacks are permitted throughout the day, that do not equal one full meal. To fast in this manner is actually quite easy once one becomes used to it, and likely has health benefits as well as spiritual.

Finally, too much eating is very harmful. Nowadays it became part of the culture, even among decent and educated people, to serve at least seven kinds of dishes; the lowest worker complains that he is disrespected when only a bowl of soup, no matter how thick and strong and deep, is served to him. And yet 2-3 bowls filled with Gsödsuppe (barley, peas and beans) nourish more than seven dishes. All these dishes definitely come together into the same stomach (no matter how many separate plates you serve and no matter how often you change knives and forks) and cause fermentation like in a pigsty; the acids attack the lining of the stomach and intestines, but the many gases penetrate the whole body, cause discomfort, often accumulate and develop disease substances, that is why an old poet wrote that Death told him that the cook hands over to him more people than wars and the plague.

The inner Cat that we all have inside us - this striving for comfort and softness- drives people to eating much meat and to eating a lot: the reason for that is comfort and mushiness. One doesn't want to walk anymore, even if one has enough time and the weather is fine; a one hour walk scares Alfred more whereas a 20 hour walk would not have scared his grandfather. People who learned how to pack sausages and wash bottles in France or Italy, or those who have one or more titles, don't want to carry any rucksack apart from an umbrella, which they mostly forget and which must not weigh more than 500 gram, nor any parcel. Carrying a rucksack is considered to be indecent; why not? Running, carrying and working stimulates digestion and thus promotes health, and goes therefore against the concept of fashion of the 20th century.

The idol of our time is a pigsty on wheels, fat, full of gas, sufficient for twenty engines, covered all over with lace, veils, pomade bottles and chocolate paper and decorated with titles of novels, which are adored by the great masses of the educated and semi-educated people who swing the censer and bend their knees, while the army of conceited, bald gentlemen, veiled ladies, dudes and pomade heroes are totally besotted.

One has to have an ideal in life, and everyone worships something, sometimes without even noticing it. If this ideal is not God, the Creator and Redeemer, then it is the absurdity in some form and thus something which kills and restricts you and causes illnesses and severe sufferings.

Meat eating, noble eating and sophisticated overeating with lots of crockery was mainly introduced by educated people. You can find a lot of sophistication in all institutes, where, in addition to a lot of knowledge, young people are also forced to adopt genteel behavior and they have to use many plates until they are also too much educated. Later on, very few people can leave behind these habits and until they reach an old age they cherish tiny cups and spoons, and want fresh tablecloths and as many plates as possible and eat large quantities like dogs from all dishes, even if there are ten of these. And those who should be role models for others because of their professional status are often the worst. It seems to us that the Lord is now about to teach those bastards to drink from large cups and be satisfied with one plate of food. There are nowhere fewer natural and perfectly reasonable people as among the educated ones. Oh happy farmers, your biggest dung heap does not stink as badly as the arrogance of the educated! There was a reason why our dear Lord wanted to be born in a stable.

Should I summarize everything in a few words and at the same time set up an unsurpassable, absolutely sure model of a healthy and sensible way of life, then I look back to Christ the Lord, who also wanted to have a human body like us, had the same natural human needs as we do (with the exception of sin) felt hunger and thirst, heat and cold, worked and became tired; Christ, our Lord is also the most perfect example of the purely natural life, the ideal of any person.

Ecce homo, what a Man! The son of the God was simple and natural in food and clothing, ate with fishermen and day laborers what they had, and could, if it was necessary, donate wine at the wedding in Cana, but he could also fast for 40 days, he was eating with Pharisees, but also making long and arduous journeys on foot, up and down, and went hungry until evening, warned in his teachings against the ruinous life of the rich, of over eating and over drinking, gave the apostles advice: "Eat what is set before you!", was so undemanding in food, drink and dwelling that he could say about himself: "The foxes have their dens and the birds their nests, but the Son of Man has nothing to put his head on."

He did not want people to be sick, but healed the sick and restored the injured nature, of course not with herbs and not with poison and not with baths, but through the divine power. But the very fact that he worked miracles to make people healthy shows that he wanted people to be healthy and that it goes against the will of God if one makes the body sick and ailing through an unreasonable way of life. Christ, the Lord, as the ideal of physical life, protects the followers of the natural healing method from craziness, from one-sidedness, from wilderness and forest devils! Therefore: Here, too, no one can lay a foundation other than that which has already been laid, that is, Jesus Christ. And whoever does not go with Him distracts.

JC: Wiser words have seldom, if ever been spoken. No one wants to do without comforts. No one wants to work hard. Yet, the simple things in life are the most important. It is the simple meals cooked by our mothers and grandmothers that are the memories we cherish, never the finest feast in a restaurant. In America, we were once fond of saying, "With freedom comes responsibility." We have at our fingertips, luxuries never dreamed of by our ancestors. Very, very few suffer from hunger in America, but millions suffer from obesity, diabetes and related diseases caused by over-consumption of unhealthy foods and lack of exercise. If we are to take control of our own health, we must use herbs, diet and modest exercise such as gardening and hiking. Fr. Kneipp insisted, "Strengthen the constitution!" Gluttony and the soft, weak, selfishness it engenders is just as distasteful now as it was in Fr. Künzle's time... we have just

become too used to it.

"Lapidar"

is a registered trademark. Legally protected from imitation. "Lapidar" consists of absolutely non-toxic plants. It causes a faster metabolism and is recommended for rheumatism, rashes, stiffness of the limbs and nervous headaches, for blood congestion and cold feet. Arteriosclerosis and varicose veins. Instructions how to use it: Adults usually take 7 to 10 tablets three times a day. Weaker or older people take a smaller amount at the beginning, which should be increased gradually. Children are given 3 to 5 tablets with honey or sugar water three times a day. The Lapidar has its full effect only if it is taken on an empty stomach, i.e. on an empty stomach or an hour before or after the meal. If there are no daily bowel movements, ask for a lapidar with the addition of Sagrada, for a weak heart with the addition of Geum. Lapidar is only real if it holds the name Joh. Künzle and is signed.

JC: I can only wonder or guess at what this might be... if anyone knows, please contact us!

Diabetes.
This nasty disease is more common than you think. The kidneys do not function well and substances such as protein and sugar, which belong in the blood, excrete with the urine. As a result, people quickly lose their strength.

And yet this disease can be fairly quickly eliminated with the use of the following herbs:
  Creeping avens (Geum alpinia/reptans/urbanum) 3 parts,

Blackberry leaves 1 part,
Blueberry leaves 1 part,
Golden five-finger herb/ dwarf yellow cinquefoil (Potentilla aurea) 2 parts,

Drink half a cup five times a day. Care should be taken to avoid all alcoholic drinks during the illness. Even later, once already healthy, you should avoid all the alcoholic drinks for a long time. Every doctor or pharmacist can diagnose this disease immediately by examining urine.
When sugar is excreted we recommend our diabetes tea A; in case of protein loss diabetes tea B. Both tea mixtures are also available in tablet form.

JC: In Fr. Künzle's time, diabetes was a much more straight forward disease. The epidemic we now face, of insulin resistance and Type 2 Diabetes was mostly unheard-of in his time. Although a dietary caused diabetes was known, especially as the British built an empire on imported sugar, the first recognized/high profile case of this modern plague was Diamond Jim Brady. Diamond Jim was financier and restaurateur with huge appetites. He is remembered as a tough, hard scrabble, "rags to riches" type, whose lavish feasts are legendary. Although, it may seem harsh or simplistic... and genetic predispositions are certainly a factor, diabetes is now almost entirely caused by diet and lifestyle. Gluttony, laziness, stress and sleep deprivation make people sick and make doctors rich. Sugar is addictive and one can develop tolerance to it. Often removing sugar from the diet has withdrawal period. Our ancestors ate very little refined sugar, and what they had was an expensive luxury. By 1900, Americans were eating 100 lbs of white sugar per year. Now, it is 160. From 1990 to 1996, diabetes increased by 40%.

Several herbs, from Prickly Pear Cactus, to Brickellia, to Dandelion, to cinnamon and even digestive bitters, help with blood sugar spikes. But, no herb or drug is effective or can replace dramatic diet and lifestyle changes. That begins with cutting out ALL refined sugar from the diet... and even fruit for some. A good friend of mine seemed almost addicted to bananas, and died of diabetes at a young age. This also means cutting out most packaged and processed foods that contain hidden sugars in the form of corn syrup... and DEFINITELY all sodas. Even "diet" soft drinks that contain aspartame affect blood sugar. A diet of meat, vegetables, natural fats and whole grains is the way to go. Avoid white bread and other "quick carbs". Alcohol consumption should be dramatically decreased or eliminated. A taste for bitter greens and sour pickles should be cultivated. Regular exercise and sufficient sleep are essential. Yes, it is difficult.... It is downright hard! Those addicted to sugar in a culture that celebrates every special event with cakes and sodas, may have a harder time quitting and reforming than a drug addict. But ask yourself, "Is this cookie worth my life?" By the way, there is no need to go overboard on the exercise. A moderately long, relaxing walk or doing 5-10 minutes jumping-jacks, push-ups or other "high intensity cardio" exercises every 2-4 hours may be just as effective in this regard as "hitting the gym."   This is yet another reason to take up gardening, as that is an exercise more rewarding and enjoyable than most!

Livestock diseases

a) severe wheezing and coughing in cattle. 1. Take 1 handful of finely chopped Masterwort (Peucedanum ostruthium), mix it with 4 handfuls of salt and give it to the cattle from time to time.

2. Take peppermint, and Anise, chop it well, sprinkle it on the food and give it to cattle.

b) Flatulence in cattle is an accumulation of gases, so that the body swells enormously. Take one or two handfuls of one of the three herbs: Fennel, Anise or Caraway, chop it up finely, boil for five minutes, it will cause winds to come out immediately and thus solves the problem.
The following recipe helps as well: simmer 1 1/2 liters of milk, crush 10 cloves of garlic and add them to the milk together with the peels, crush 1 tablespoon full of Caraway and 1 spoonful of pepper and give it warm.

"Against the fullness in cattle, we usually use the following: Heat about 1 - 1 1/2 liters of milk, add about 10 crushed garlic cloves with peels, add a spoonful of caraway and pepper and give the warm liquid to the cattle. It is a very good remedy and we repeat the same every year." (a letter from a farmer)

c) Diarrhea and "calf paralysis". Give it generously dried Lady's Mantle to eat; this will help soon.
Fever of pregnant cows. Simmer Meadowsweet and give it to the cow to drink.

d) Stomach cold. Two to three handfuls of juniper berries with peppermint.

e) General malaise if one does not quite know what is wrong. Simmer peppermints and juniper berries and cumin and give this to the cattle repeatedly; afterwards a big amount of dried nettles. Cattle eat it greedily, it helps in such cases.

f) Lumps without pus will quickly disappear if you apply crushed ferns or you simmer ferns with vinegar and then rub them in.

g) Lumps with pus. Boil herbal hay and make a poultice. Mountain flowers hay from nutrient-poor meadows are always more effective than herbal hay from nutrient-rich meadows.

h) Inflammation of the eyes, mouth, throat, etc. Crush Herb Robert (geranium robertianum) and apply; ferns help too.

i) Erysipele (an infectious disease caused by the bacterium Erysipelothrix rhusiopathiae) in pigs. Collect a lot of moss from stones, roofs, from the forest, if possible damp, place the pig on it and cover it with moss; it takes away the inflammation. If you can instill St John's wort oil, it is even better (or castor oil).

Foot and mouth disease

I don't know any absolutely safe preventive agent. On the other hand, I am aware of many recent cases where farmers have completely cured very large cowsheds of contaminated cattle in a period of 8 to 14 days.

a) The cattle are given 1 to 2 liters of thyme or marjoram tea several times a day, and the hooves are also washed with it.

b) The cattle are given a tablespoon full of masterwort with a little salt three times a day, and masterwort is boiled in water and the hooves are washed with the liquid.

c) In both cases the kidney area of the animals is rubbed vigorously several times a day with grated raw onions, for this is usually the place where the disease sits.

JC: The use of herbs in veterinary conditions is beyond my experience, although the old folks in the mountains where I

grew up had a very similar tradition of using herbs in that way. I have no reason to doubt that Fr. Künzle's advice in this regard is equally valid.

Appendicitis
is sometimes quickly eased by blackberry leaves or holly tea and an immediate application of Milanese plasters. In any case, call the doctor immediately.

JC: Fr. Künzle's advice to "call the doctor immediately" cannot be stated too strongly in cases of appendicitis. The symptoms of this disease are often mistaken as arising from another cause and the patient waits too long for a doctor's help. The consequences of which can be deadly.

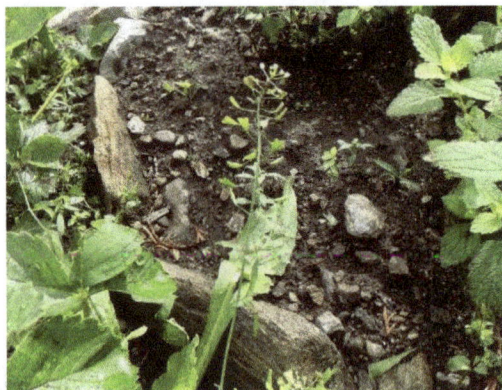
Shepherd's Purse

(Bleeding nose) Epistaxis

stops almost immediately when you tie a handful of fresh shepherd's purse (Capsella bursa pastoris) around the bleeding person's neck. If shepherd's purse is not at hand, do the same with a handful of fresh grass; if the bleeding occurs frequently, only hawkweed with egg will help.

JC: Many styptic and astringent herbs, such as Yarrow, are good for nose bleed, but Fr. Künzle's remedies are certainly more pleasant than some... such as cayenne pepper or cinnamon!

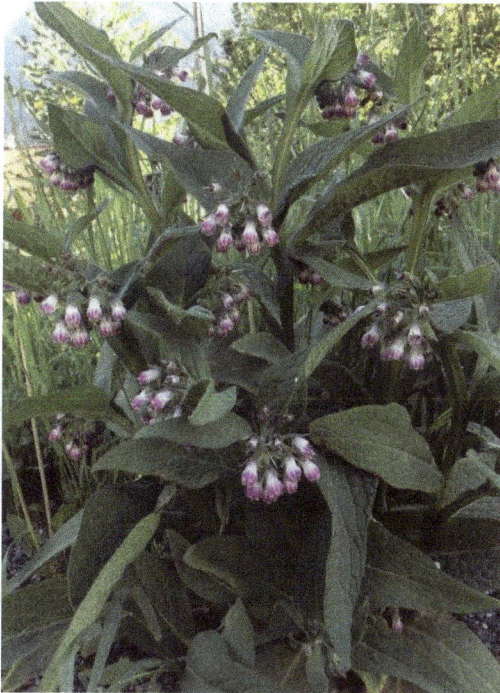

Comfrey

Healing ointment.

In response to multiple requests, I am publishing here a recipe for the preparation of a healing ointment. The following herbs, individually or mixed, are required:

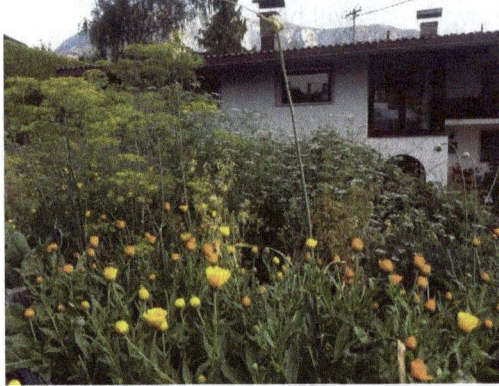

Pot Marigold

St. John's wort, yarrow leaves, marigolds, plantain, kidney vetch, comfrey, arnica, lady's mantle, sanicle, Pimpinella, Meadowsweet. These herbs are crushed, if possible fresh, boiled with lard for 3-4 hours, the liquid lard is then strained through a cloth; as soon as it cools down, the ointment is ready.

This ointment, which is produced by us under the name of Anthyllis Healing Ointment, is good for all cuts, wounds and grazes that need to heal. However, is not suitable as a cooling ointment.

JC: This is an excellent ointment. There is little doubt that this astringent, anti-inflammatory, calming and bruise dispersing concoction would be good for many complaints.

Schwini, Schwund,

is the name given to the shortening or thinning of an arm or foot; sometimes it gets painful, sometimes it is painless. If it is painless, it can be healed by pouring cold water over the affected limb several times a day for 4-6 weeks and then rubbing it thoroughly from top down. However, if the Schwini is painful, then it is connected with rheumatism; in this case, cold water will do only harm. Then rub the relevant limb several times a day with the following mixture:

take a handful of Lady's Mantle and a handful of shepherd's purse, pour good brandy or the first run of Brandy onto them, cover it well and expose it to the heat of the sun or stove for 10-14 days; then strain the liquid. Rubbing it in several times a day helps in most cases. Available under the name "Krafttropfen Robur".

JC: In Fr. Künzle's time, such maladies would likely be caused by polio or tuberculosis. But, withering or atrophy can be a result of injury or other causes. Hopefully an open minded physical therapist will make use of this advice and report back to us on its effectiveness.

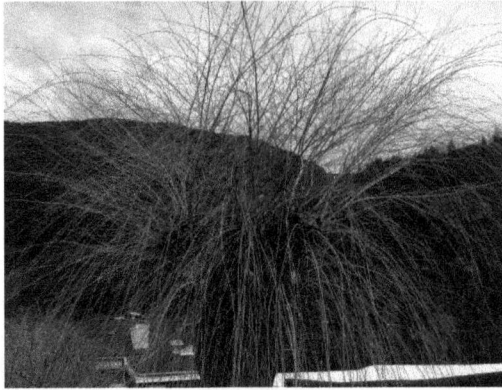

Willow

Weak legs.

Old people whose legs are weak, because of old age or because of an illness could strengthen their legs in frequent foot baths in boiled willow bark. The basket weavers sell bark cheaply.

JC: Willow Bark was the original source of salicylic acid, the precursor to aspirin. Such a soak would reduce inflammation and pain. It would also help with callouses, hard skin, thickened toenails and cracked heels. It would tonify the skin and generally make the legs and feet more comfortable.

Tea making rules.

All teas work best when you take a spoonful every hour.

Unless specifically stated otherwise, the herbs should be boiled, not just blanched. Alpine herbs require longer boiling times than valley herbs. Root tea needs one to two hours of boiling.
Sugar may be added anywhere unless the opposite is stated, but

the effect is greater where no sugar is used. Brown, yellow and black sugar is better than the white one.

How many herbs and how much water? No precise quantities can be determined here; if you take more herbs, the drink becomes stronger. Only with poisonous plants one has to be very careful; however, these should and may only be prescribed by the doctor; actually, in this little book we have presented lots of non-toxic herbs for internal use.

JC: Jolanta and I agree that this is where we differ with Fr. Künzle. Boiling is good in making a decoction of herbal roots. But, for leaves and flowers, it is best to preserve the volatile oils that would evaporate with boiling. Pouring boiling water over the herbs, and covering the vessel while the herbs steep, results in a more potent infusion.

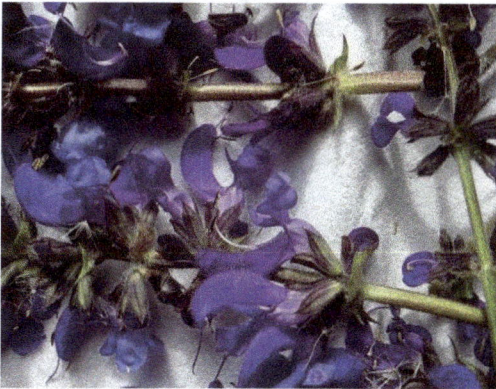

Meadow Sage

Tea for flu

A sip of a mixture of a handful of wormwood, a handful of sage, a handful of Alpine speedwell, a handful of liquorice every morning and evening, protects against flu. Those who are already ill with flu take a spoonful every half an hour and recover in two days.

JC: Fr. Künzle was remarkably prescient in giving this advice. Not long after his writings, which were not translated into English (likely due to the World Wars) a flu epidemic ravished America and much of the western world, with results that make COVID-19 seem mild. The most effective treatment found was a variety of the artemisia family, the wormwoods. Unfortunately, this discovery has been overlooked by modern medicine... perhaps, because pharmaceutical drugs have far more potential to generate revenue than a plant given to us freely by God. Herbalists need not be ignorant to the cures that grow beneath our feet. By law, we cannot officially recommend an herb for the stated purpose of curing or treating any health condition... even, if it would save millions of lives. All we can say, whether in this use of artemisia or any other advice given in this book is, that the herbs have been historically used for this purpose and that Fr. Künzle recommended them. Fr. Künzle, himself had to fight legal battles with the medical establishment and government regulators in his day. Fortunately for all of humanity, he prevailed!

Tea for children.

When children have a fever, rashes, sores, severe itching, are always pale and tired, it is mostly the problem of the kidneys; as soon as this kidney catarrh is gone, it is followed by excessive urine excretion, the healing often comes in a day. For this we need Couch Grass and some mint; if there is also constipation, add fennel powder. Available ready-to-use under the name of Pastor Künzles "Kindertee".

JC: Fevers in children can often come on very quickly and are much more dangerous than comparable fevers in adults. Children should be closely monitored, and medical treatment sought immediately if the fever threatens to go too high.

Contagious diseases.

When typhoid, cholera and other epidemics are around, one uses garlic or half a teaspoon of Burnet saxifrage, or Masterwort root powder, or garden Angelica root powder in cider, wine or milk every day. The roots are cut up and dried very well and then ground in the coffee grinder. These substances destroy a lot of germs.

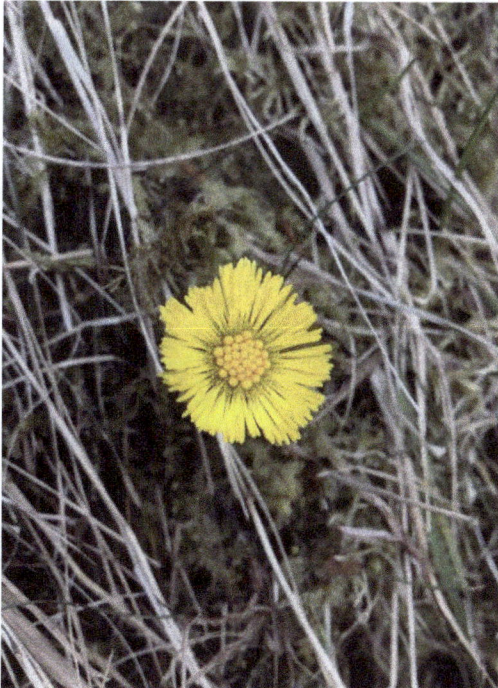

Coltsfoot

If the plague is about, which God may graciously prevent, one should collect coltsfoot or butterbur (Tussilago, Petasites); this is the root of a large mountain butterbur, the leaves of which are often 50 cm in diameter, green above and white below. The roots must be well dried and then powdered; when eaten, they cause strong sweating; only those who can sweat excessively will be healed.

Flu.

This disease takes hold of everything: the nerves of the head, kidneys, bladder, lungs, and often the heart and the stomach. Our flu tea brings relief. The patient is given a sip every hour. The main thing is that a lot of urine is excreted; if this is not the case, despite drinking the flu tea, then watch out. It means that the kidneys stopped working; a simple remedy can help here. Take two onions or two garlic, crush them and place them raw on both kidneys and leave them there for 3-7 hours; the kidneys start working again and a lot of urine comes out. Then the flu cannot develop into pneumonia.

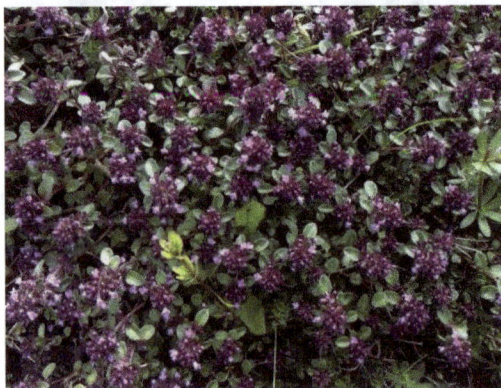
Thyme

Aftereffects of the flu.

Many people have not felt well since they had flu. Some excrete too little urine when compared to before and they need onions and garlic as described above. Others have a weak heart; for those I advise my mixture with Creeping avens (Geum). Others have lost their appetite; for those I advise my stomach powder, also available in tablet form. Others feel weak and have no life energy; for them I advise my basic herbal mixture (Lapidar)

JC: The use of herbal antiseptics and antibiotics is very old, and generally does include garlic. Garlic and all of the allium family are powerful herbs. Legend has it that when the Black Plague was devastating Europe, a group of thieves prospered by robbing the houses of those who had recently died of the disease. When finally apprehended and tried, they were forced to admit to authorities how they were able to avoid infection. The concoction became known as "Four Thieves Tonic", and although there are many variations, it is a mixture of garlic and herbs in raw vinegar. This tonic is so effective that several attempts have been made to patent it in both American and Canada. So far, folk medicine has won out against business interests. "Fire Cider" is another variant on the concept. Recipes for both Four Thieves and Fire Cider abound on the internet and in books, so the reader may find those that suit their needs in other resources. During cold and flu season, this author has found a daily regimen of garlic, oil of oregano, turmeric, thyme and black pepper, along with plenty of fermented pickles and peppers, along with supplemental vitamin C, zinc and vitamin D to be beneficial.

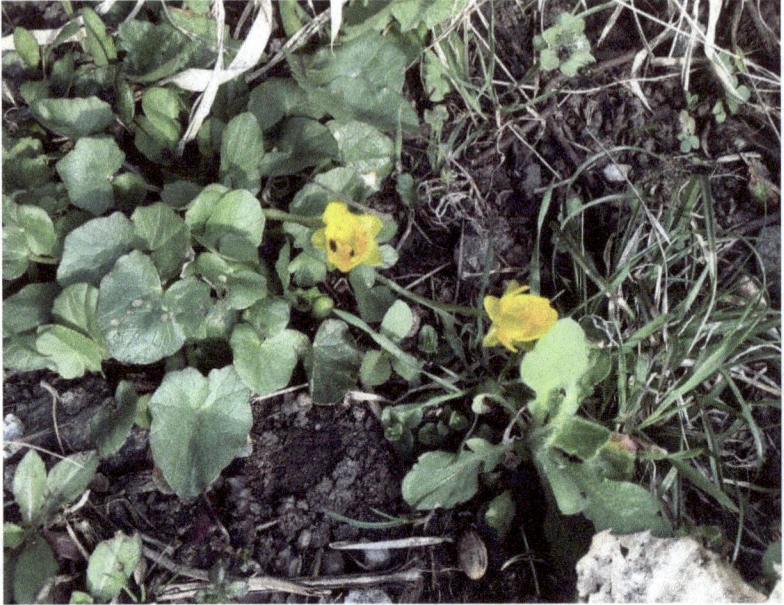

Lesser Celandine

She was called Wart Bethli,

because both of her hands were full of warts. A teacher once jokingly called her so and the nickname has stayed with her to this day, although for 50 years she has had no more warts; but since then she has found out a lot about remedies for this decoration; whoever has them and wants to get rid of them goes to her; but I am not allowed to reveal her place of residence, she would not have liked that.

How did she get rid of this ornament? She followed the advice of a Capuchin to whom she went for advice, she dabbed these warts three times a day with a little bit of garlic juice; after 8 days they were all gone. She gave this advice to many. Others, who had their hands full, were instructed to fix chopped onions every night; usually the warts disappeared after only 5 nights. In the summer time she usually gave celandine or milkweed to the children with warts. They had to dab the raised areas several times for a few days, and then the warts disappeared.

But I know a herdsman who lives in Appenzell, who would simply run his hands over them and mutter a few words; after a few days the warts will be gone; is that magic? No, it is just the magnetic power of these people; muttering certain words only increases confidence and then it has the effect of self persuasion.

JC: The latex or sap from dandelion stems applied regularly to warts, has also been found by many to be useful in their removal.

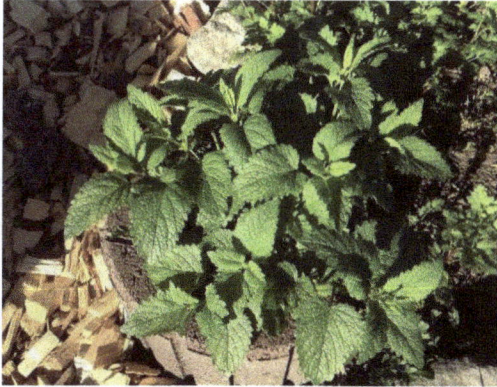

Lemon Balm

For old people

sleep is important, because during sleep the blood is detoxified from many harmful substances; if you don't sleep, then all kinds of disease substances develop and from them many disturbances arise. A glass of good wine in the evening helps many to fall asleep, while others achieve the same with a warm foot bath. Many sleep well if they place a crushed, slightly warmed onion or garlic under the back of their head. Others drink a cup of lemon balm tea. Many people fall asleep easily if they dip a pair of socks in hot vinegar, wring them out, put them on and then pull a couple of woolen socks over them and go to bed with them.

The second important condition for old people is proper bowel movements and urination; without these two things either they die soon or continue living in misery and pain. "Young people can die, but everyone must die," is the saying. Death is nothing terrible for believing Christians, it is not an actual death at all, but a transition to immortality and to eternal youth.

Old people often have peculiarities, but young people usually have more; one should take these peculiarities into account and be patient, because this brings reward when one is old oneself.

JC: Another "remedy" used in German Folk Medicine, that has proved quite effective for many, is to make a small pillow or sachet of dried hops flowers. These are placed by or on the pillow in one's bed to induce sleep. It is said that in the days of hand picking, workers often fell asleep while working on hops farms.

The wine maker from Winital

had his own extensive vineyard and served only his own wine. The last wine in the barrel, however, was of a lower quality, as everywhere, and for the sake of his reputation he did not want to serve it. He made it into vinegar and knew how to use it even better than the wine; for he used it as a remedy.

The head teacher from the same area was often suffering from severe cold. The wine maker advised him to boil a liter of vinegar and a liter of water in the pot; as soon as it was hot, the teacher had to hold his head over it and put a thick cloth over his head and over the pot so that all the steam could rise to his head for about a quarter of an hour; then the cold was gone.

In case of bronchial catarrh, the same procedure had to be repeated twice a day, the only difference being that the chest also had to be uncovered; in three days the catarrh was gone.
People with weak lungs, predispositions to pulmonary consumption and tuberculosis were advised by our wine maker to put 3-5 flat plates with vinegar in the bedroom every evening. The smell of the vinegar that was inhaled all night refreshed and strengthened the lungs to such an extent that after a year people became very healthy again. With advanced tuberculosis, however, this remedy could no longer cure. The wine maker found out this method through a relative of his, who ran a vinegar factory with 200-300 workers, none of whom had any lung problems. He also employed people with tuberculosis, and they all recovered.

The old town councilor complained to the wine maker that he always had a bad itching in bed and had to scratch, which was usually followed by a burning skin during the day. "It's easy to help here," laughed the wine maker, "put a bowl with vinegar and a sponge in your bedroom and wash your itchy places with it, do this every evening, and you will have peace." He did that and really found peace.

As his wife saw that, she wanted to know whether the winemaker knew a remedy against dandruff. He also gave her useful advice: "Take two tablespoons full of vinegar and ten tablespoons of warm water and wash and rub your head with it daily, and the dandruff will disappear". "But," was the anxious question, "doesn't it harm hair growth?" "On the contrary, the hair will be much thicker." Here too, the winemaker was brilliantly right.

The winemaker also had frequent visits from cyclists who had suffered sprains or bruises from falling or bumping. He advised them to use his vinegar; they had to constantly put vinegar poultices on injured places, which resulted in being cured usually in 10-15 hours.

The road worker Sepp suffered from pain in his wrists and in his big toe and could no longer work. He who would otherwise avoid going to pubs, this time turned to the winemaker and told him about his suffering. He cured him in the following way: he dipped a napkin , folded four times into hot vinegar and placed it on the affected area and repeated this procedure every time the napkin got cold; after 24 hours all the pain was gone and road worker was back to work again.

The sawmill worker Lunzi suffered terribly from lumbago in his back and could neither stand nor walk and lay in bed like a piece of wood; his wife ran to the wine maker, told him, while weeping, what had happened and returned with a bottle of vinegar. She warmed it, took a linen towel, folded it eight times, dipped it into warm vinegar, placed it on the painful area and put a dry, woolen cloth over it. The pain was gone after a few hours.

JC: Vinegar has countless healthful applications! The key is in getting good quality, raw vinegar. When buying vinegar, look for the terms, "raw", "unfiltered", Unpasteurized" and the questionable term, "organic." Organic was once the Gold Standard by which natural foods were judged, but business interest and government corruption have rendered it almost meaningless... too often, the "organic" product is of poorer quality and the use of fertilizers, pesticides, etc in its growth and

production are just as bad as the less expensive, fresher, non-organic produce in the next bin. Organic has become a marketing ploy and bureaucracy. If you do buy your vinegar, try to find a bottle with a "mother" in it. The vinegar mother is a formation of the vinegar bacteria that not only proves your vinegar is alive but can be used to make your own vinegar! The best of most anything is always that which you make yourself!

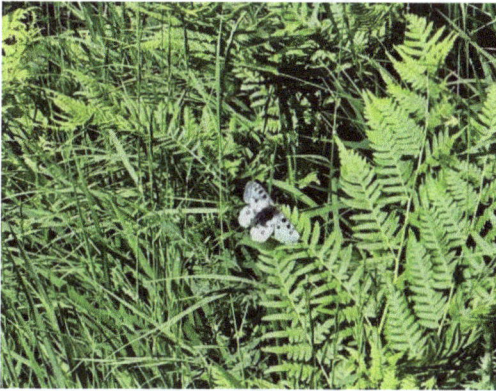

Fern

The ferns

 belong to the most delicate and useful plants. There are several thousand species, from the small wall fern to the giant tree fern growing in warm countries; they compete with palm trees with the splendour of their leaves, yes there are ferns whose leaves are five meters long. In coal mines one can find fern trunks thick like full-grown fir trees; these are the giant ferns of prehistoric times. All kinds of ferns are beneficial for rheumatism, used either as an underlay for sleeping or for full baths or foot baths; the mountain ferns, however, are much stronger than those of the plains. Furthermore, all kinds of ferns are worm-resistant; all kinds of flies, horseflies and worms avoid ferns; an old legend tells us that even the devil frowns and pulls a wry face every time he passes a fern, just like a truant from school does, when he walks past the schoolhouse. The large wood fern (Filix mas) is still used as a tapeworm remedy; the small ferns such as the wall fern, the Southern maidenhair fern, Hart's tongue fern, the fountain fern can safely be used internally as tea against worms.

The fern is of great benefit to mountaineers, especially when going downhill. Many then put fresh fern into their shoes, which takes away the tiredness; others tie ferns around their knees, which removes the dreaded meniscus problems, others fill both trouser pockets and pockets in the heart area with fern and claim that this helps them to walk much more easily. Forest workers who spend the night in barracks and cannot find hay or straw anywhere to camp for the night, make a bed of green ferns and have a safe rest on them. If you suddenly start feeling rheumatism in your knees or heels and can hardly go any further, tie green fern to the painful areas and you will be able to walk again after 5 minutes.

The strength of the large forest fern root is noticeably great in case of foot or calf cramps in bed; if you put such a root on your feet, the cramp disappears; the same root retains this power for two years.

Thus the Creator (who else?) put these healing powers in the fern.

JC: I think my biggest take away, or lesson from Fr. Künzle's book is the wealth of benefits offered by the ferns. In fact, I have been so impressed by his teaching on this subject as to have purchased several books on identifying ferns in the wild, propagating and growing ferns. I hope our readers will do the same!

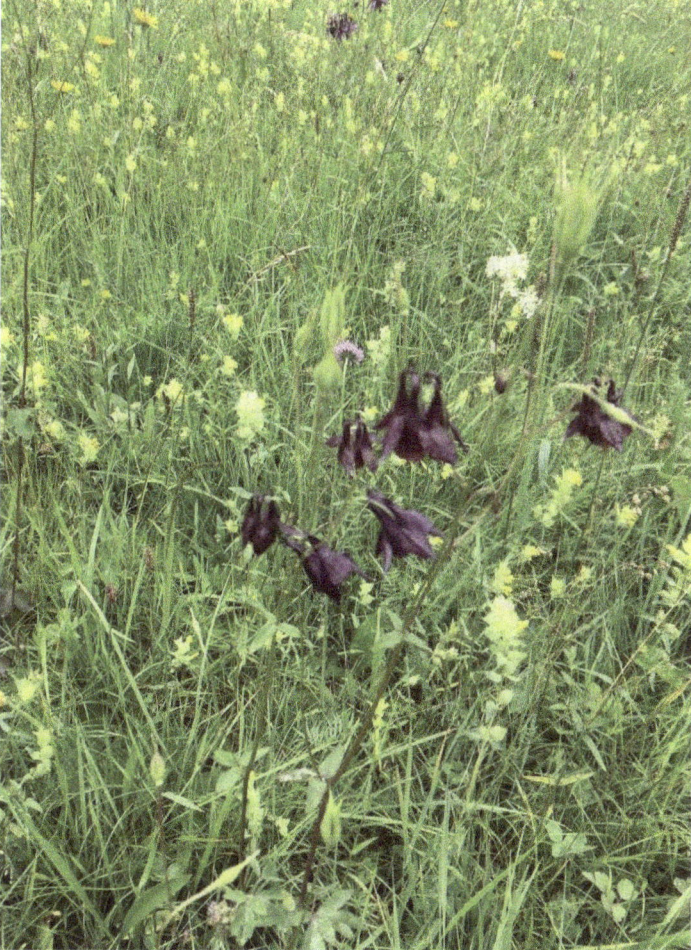

Columbine

The buttercups species and their use.

Everybody knows the creeping buttercup (Ranunculus) with its 5 golden petals like everybody knows the tax collector, and it is as unpopular as the tax collector; the cattle don't like it either and leave it to grow; and yet it is very useful to the meadows; the grass in the meadows where buttercup grows is considerably stronger than without it; the gloriously radiant blossoms of this weed reflect the light back onto the surrounding grass, and so give the grass more strength. The yellow buttercup species have strength in their roots which draws out blisters; I knew a man who suffered a lot from gout. This man who had been in bed for over a year and who cured himself with buttercups roots by crushing them and applying them on the affected areas; soon large blisters formed, which he pierced, whereupon the substance of the disease ran out and the pain subsided. Onion poultices would have done the same and with much less pain.

The white buttercup (the common water-crowfoot) that grows in wet meadows is a wonderful ornamental plant and has a very pleasant smell and is called Magdalena flower by the country folk because it is usually to be found in beautiful bloom during their festival in July. Those who make a pilgrimage to Einsiedeln via the mountain Etzel in July will find this flower in great quantities.

The lovely anemones belong to this family. The white buttercups can be found in large quantities in sunny, poor-nutrient meadows and on the edges of forests and in forest clearings; internally it is not used because of its sharpness; it is used, however, externally against freckles by putting the flower into alcohol and then you can wash the face with this tincture.

The blue anemone (Anemone hepatica) known as hepatica, which has beautiful leaves nicely formed in three parts, is more widely used; they are used for jaundice and liver diseases of all kinds, and can be found in our liver tea. The gardeners plant the wonderful garden anemone De Caen, which requires a dry and sunny place.

The yellow marsh marigold (Caltha palustris) also belongs to this family; they are also called Easter flowers and are used to dye Easter eggs. The ancients saw in the five large golden leaves an image of the risen Savior and his five wounds.

The Columbine (Aquilegia) thrives on sunny, nutrient poor meadows and is grown in gardens in all colors. Herbs and blossoms are beneficial for all liver ailments and edema; they are boiled in red wine and afterwards the wine is strained and kept in bottles. The patients take a sip of it in the morning on an empty stomach and in the evening before going to bed. The same potion is also used to strengthen the heart.

The meadow star (Ficaria verna) is a very lovely small plant and can be found in damp meadows. The yellow flower resembles a star. The whole plant is used only externally as poultice for gout and rheumatism by drawing blisters like buttercup, but only when you use it fresh; it also heals hemorrhoid ulcers when applied to them.

Our well-known old man's beard (Clematis vitalba), these graceful climbing plants, also belong to this group. They tend to creep up to the top of the trees and form a wonderful ornament with their white flowers in the summer and with their large, white, woolly seed heads in autumn. The country folk use the tough herb to make wreaths, for supporting tree branches and the like; the boys make their first attempts and smoke the hollow, dry stalks. "Old man's beard" leaves freshly placed in the shoes and walked on them all day alleviate the gout pain and heal the corns.

JC: Of the flowers Fr. Künzle mentions above, the most often used by modern herbalists is the Anemone. This herb has a remarkable use in certain mental states such as panic attacks,

anxieties relating to Post Traumatic Stress, calming an enraged person or even affecting one in a fugue state. The tincture is strong and can be irritating. It should only be used by one who has thoroughly learned its use, so I leave this as a suggestion to our readers for further study. As for the blistering effects of Buttercups... I will stick with Fr. Künzle's advice to use onions instead!

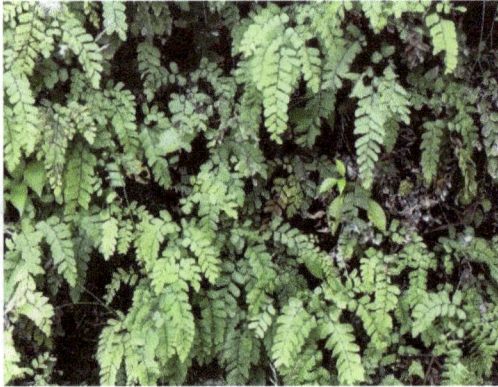

Lumbago

is a sudden painful inflammation of the muscles of the spine. A forest worker who was hit by it, needed three hours to reach home, but he could hardly walk, collected a bunch of fern leaves and stuffed them onto the affected area, whereupon after a quarter of an hour he was able to walk again and lost all pain as he walked. Another time, when there was no fern nearby, he managed almost as well with moss; a third time, when there was no moss around, he put a lump of damp earth on it with good success.

A bricklayer, who suffered from lumbago quite often, managed to get away with a very warm cloth over the affected area;

another time he heated sand, tied two handfuls in his handkerchief and placed it onto the painful area.

- A farmer managed to help himself by crushing 2-3 garlic and placing it on the hurting spot.

- - A carpenter suffered terribly from lumbago. The man had a very urgent order and could not possibly wait long without serious problems; an old colleague who visited him advised him to chop up fern roots and lie with his back on them; he did that, his colleague got roots for him. After three days, he was healed and returned to work.

A blacksmith used to flagellate the painful area of lumbago with a bunch of fresh nettles, after which the skin got covered with red spots full of disease substance; these spots burned a lot, so he put fresh coltsfoot leaves on to calm the burn.

JC: Once again, we learn of the power of ferns! Jolanta has mentioned using moss to treat her husband.. Garlic may well be as close to a panacea as God has ever provided. In this instance, Stinging Nettles are being used as a "counter irritant", however, the "venom" of the sting is much like that of bee venom which is used by many for inflammation and pain.

A final reflection from Fr. Künzle:

The Laplander in the Park of Copenhagen and the deciduous trees.

Not long ago, a famous and wealthy Dane brought a young Laplander from the icy north to Copenhagen. The boy who had never seen a tree was like in heaven for the splendor of the never-seen trees in the city park. "What kind of tree is that?" he asked, pointing to a 40 meter high poplar. The Dane told him that there were hundreds of thousands of such trees and many species, and showed him the beautiful white poplar and explained to him that these trees were very elastic, the storm wind would not break them, but they would break the wind and are, therefore, planted in long rows along streets and channels; their wood is the best against moisture; they hold and drain the soil, and high above the birds nest.

At the town pond, the Laplander noticed an old willow, so thick in diameter, that the trunk could not be spanned by him and the Dane together. "What kind of tree is that?" "Listen, without the willows, of which there are more than you have ice floes, we would have no baskets, no wickerwork, no wreaths. Many people live on wickerwork, the farmers plant them by the water and need the branches to bind all kinds of smaller plants and to strengthen their fences; these willows thrive wherever it is damp, up to the mountains, and hold the ground so that the avalanches and brooks do not wash it away.

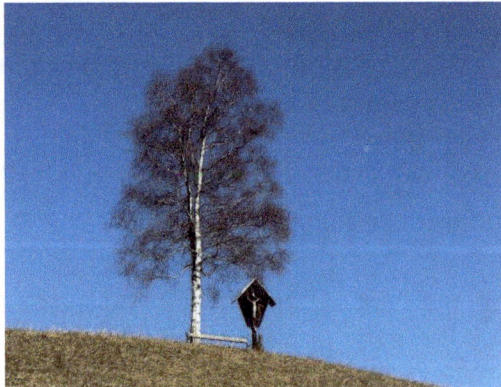

Birch Tree

The man from icy land particularly liked the birch with its fine, delicate foliage, which playfully moved in the wind. The Dane explained to him that there are forests full of birch where it is very healthy to sojourn, the leaves are a delicious medicine for urine ailments, the sap of the tree is a useful drink against edema.

On the other bank of the city pond, the laplander noticed alder bushes. "What are they for?" This is the most undemanding tree; it grows by millions where there is water, grows quickly, if it is cut down, it regrows twice as much as before; it holds the ground of the banks, so that the water does not carry it away and drains the soil so that it does not turn into a swamp; without alders, vast, magnificent plains would be only swamps and gravel.

As he walked on, the guest from the north noticed a hazelnut bush full of nuts. This is the joy and sometimes this also causes the suffering of our boys. The boys collect the nuts and they taste wonderful; but if the boys behave badly, the father takes a rod from this bush and beats the boys; and also mothers who want to keep the house tidy keep such a rod like this in the parlour behind the mirror.

The young man was astonished and in awe when he saw seven mighty beeches in all their splendid foliage. "You see, you can walk for hours in the forests of these trees, they give wonderful fresh air, provide strong wood for joiners and carpenters and wonderful heating material; millions have work and bread and warmth thanks to it. In autumn it is full of small, oily nuts, which many forest animals feed on; look up there, the birds build nests and here leaps a squirrel from branch to branch.

A bit further inside, the boy saw a couple of tall old oaks of a mighty girth and not less than forty meters high. The Dane explained to him: "It is the strongest of all our trees, solid as iron, its wood is extremely valued and expensive; without the oak you would not have been able to travel by train, because the sleepers on which the rails are fastened are made of oak. Our carpenters make the most durable and most expensive furniture out of it. When he plucked an acorn for the boy, the latter was astounded: "That looks like my father's tobacco pipe; Oh how nice, I'll take it home with me." The Dane explained to him that these acorns make healthy coffee, in Hungary they are used to fatten the pigs; the pagans considered these trees sacred and regarded them as the seat of the gods.

Higher up there was a tall, old chestnut tree with fruits covered in prickly pods. The laplander was beside himself from surprise when the Dane opened the shell and showed him the fruit. "This tree provides food for millions of people because these fruits are extremely nutritious." "But why are these spikes all around?" Without this protection birds and squirrels and insects would eat everything up; the almighty Creator added this protective skin; when the fruit is ripe, it falls to the ground, the protective cover pops up and we can collect it. In the south they have even much taller trees; near the fire-spitting mountain Etna there is a chestnut tree under which 200 riders and their horses have enough space.

Now they came to an old walnut tree that was full of fruit. The Dane showed him a couple of nuts, which he took out of his pocket, crushed them and handed them to the boy; how he liked them! "Look! These fruits grow on this tree; the further you go to the south, the more there are such trees; they are very precious; the wood is very beautiful and makes wonderful furniture, the fresh leaves are beneficial to those who use them for headache; the boiled leaves cleanse the blood, the fruits, as you can see, are delicious and nutritious.

"But where did you get all these trees from, who made them?"
"The one who created the earth and the sun and the sea."
"You are then certainly very grateful to him?"
"Grateful? No, there is no gratitude among people!"

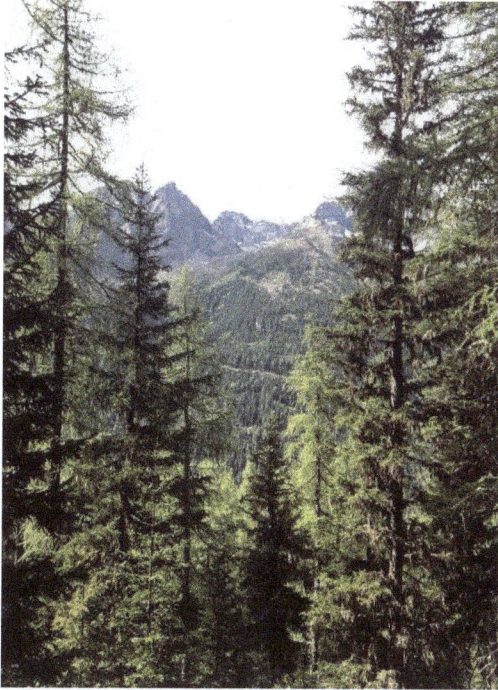

JW: Trees

For us - herbalists, herbal teachers - all plants: trees, bushes, shrubs, moss, lichen, flowers, herbs, whether wild or cultural, whether full of scent or simple grass ... they are all herbs full of wonderful, mysterious, healing, spiritual, nutritious, energetic powers.

This part of the book introduces trees and their roles in people's life. Trees provide oxygen, humidity, shade in the heat, cover in the rain, they stop erosion of banks and shores, they keep mountain slopes from sliding down, they are home to so many animals and birds.... and, apart from all that and many other things they are our food and medicine.

Trees definitely are my source of health and energy and I would like to share my experience in how certain trees are being used in my region.

Poplar
Poplar bud tincture is highly valued in our region. Maybe because poplar is a rare tree here. Trees protect their buds with resin. Bees know that. They have been collecting resin from the buds for thousands of years and have been turning it into propolis - the highly protective, antibacterial, antiviral, antifungal substance with which they protect and disinfect their beehive. We, humans, most probably have learned that from the bees, but, as we cannot turn it into Propolis with our bodies, like bees do, we make tinctures.

I collect some buds and with the help of high percentage Alcohol I get the resin from them and turn it into tincture. Diluted internally it is used for inflammations, colds, flu; externally for rashes, small wounds, muscle pain. I use it for gurgling when I feel that I might develop a sore throat.

Since I have bees, I have stopped collecting poplar buds. Instead, I take a little bit of Propolis from my bee hives, turn it into tincture and use it in the same way as poplar bud tincture. I like toothpaste with Propolis. It does so much more than just cleaning the teeth.

Willow
Willow bark together with Meadowsweet is part of Bayer
Aspirin. As I am always careful to have enough willow bark and
Meadowsweet at home, I use only my homemade "Aspirin".
In spring, just before the buds start opening I cut a few two or
three year old twigs from a willow. The twigs are thinner than
the thickness of a finger. I peel the bark, cut it into 1 cm pieces,
dry it well and store it in tightly closed dark jars or in a dark
place.

Whenever I have fever, flu, pains in joints or muscles or a
headache, I make a decoction/infusion: I soak 1 spoon of
powdered willow bark in 1 Liter of cold water for half an hour,
then heat it on a very low heat for another 20-30 minutes, but
do not bring it to a boil. I add a spoon of dried meadowsweet
and I might add some lemon verbena or lemon balm or lavender
for a better taste and a better sleep. I let the infusion soak for 10
minutes, strain it, pour into thermos and drink half a cup or a
cup every three, four hours. I know, I have to wait for the
soothing effect of the remedy, as it has to pass through the
"chemical factory" of my body before the healing substances of
the plants start to work, but then the healing powers start
working.

A quicker version is making an infusion: pour 500 ml of very hot,
but not boiling water onto 1 teaspoon of powdered willow bark
and 1 teaspoon of powdered meadow sweet, leave 15 minutes
to draw and drink many times a day.

Well, this is my way of getting rid of infections with fever
without ruining my stomach.

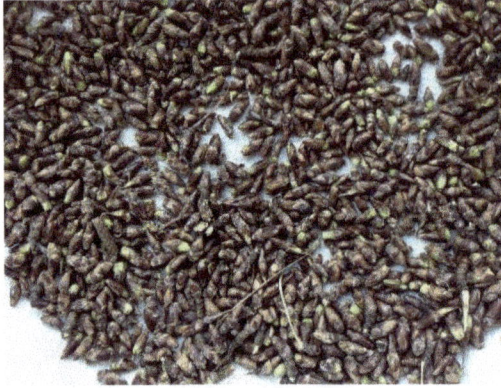

Birch Buds

Birch

I love birch trees. They are so beautiful with their white trunks and the shade they cast is light, shivering of the leaves in the light breeze on a hot summer day. It is a very robust tree. A pioneer tree - one of the first ones to start growing after avalanches, mud slides, volcano eruptions.

Birch is so generous and we are given so much from the birch: sap, buds, leaves. Sap is my favorite. Every second spring I am waiting for that moment, when I can drill a small hole into the body of my birch, insert a straw into it and then enjoy the sap - cold, slightly sweet. I take a few Liters from the tree during a period of 5-7 days and then I close the hole, so that the leaves have enough water and minerals.

My day's portion is about 50 Grams on an empty stomach as I want to get the most of it. The rest I keep in the fridge. It would stay fresh for a day, but then it starts fermenting. I freeze the rest - it will be for the next year, when I do not exploit my tree.

I use birch water for boosting my immune system, for more energy, which I sometimes lack in spring. Birch water has many useful minerals. It is also used for the skin and hair. Every man in German speaking countries would know birch water against hair loss and dandruff.

I collect birch buds round the same time, when I enjoy sap. The right time is when the tops of the buds turn green. I cut a few twigs, dry them, brush off the buds, powder them in a coffee grinder and store them in a jar. The powdered buds land on my salad, soup, on bread or are added to my morning herbal infusion. I use the buds for strengthening my immune system, for detoxification.

And then come the soft spring leaves. They are part of my salad, or I just eat a few leaves now and then when I pass a birch tree.

Towards summer, I collect birch leaves - the young and healthy ones. These I dry for my detox mixtures (they are mild diuretic) and for anti-inflammatory mixtures. And then I leave my birch in peace, until next spring.

Hazelnut
When I think of a hazelnut, I think of nuts. One does not have to introduce them. I eat a lot of nuts. I believe that nuts give me a lot of energy, they are full of vitamins and minerals, thus it is my super food when I go on long hikes.

I eat them raw, as any roasting, baking, cooking will destroy part of the valuable properties. If one has problems with digesting nuts - this is my advice. Soak a handful of nuts in cold water, keep them for the night and eat them during the next day. The nuts will be much lighter to digest, but they will still have all their valuable ingredients inside. Unfortunately, the number of allergic people is increasing, so be sure that you are not allergic before you consume nuts.

Leaves are also valuable. I like the young ones and add them to my spring and early summer salads.

Beech
I admire these mighty trees. They are so majestic, and they have very cute offsprings. Have you ever seen the young shoots of a beech? No? Look out for these. You will definitely enjoy the look of them. And have you ever eaten the nuts of a beech? My grandson introduced me to these. We do not have beeches in the Alps, but he lives next to huge beech forests. In autumn the paths are strewn with burrs - those tiny boxes with beech nuts. My grandson showed me how to open them with scissors. Just cutting the pointed upper part and then peeling the seed. Mmmmm delicious!

A beech gives not only nuts. I have read that one huge beech tree releases per hour enough oxygen for 50 people to breath during that hour. We do need such trees!

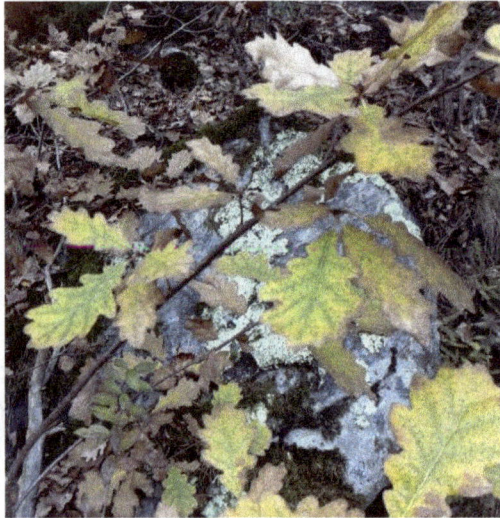

Oak

Oak bark is my strongest anti-inflammatory, antiseptic home medicine. I always have oak bark at home, but, thank God, I very seldom need it. I collect oak bark in the same way as I collect willow bark and keep it dried in a jar. I would use oak bark decoction externally for washing the wounds which do not heal properly, or for very strong perspiration of the feet, although, after what I have read in this book, I might never "heal" sweaty feet. As sweat bodies detoxify themselves, so why hem this process?

I might use oak bark decoction for a very severe diarrhea, but, so far, I have not done that, as I have never had one. Well, it is very important to know the reason for diarrhea, especially when it is severe, thus consulting a doctor is always useful.

I use oak leaves in my recipe for fermented cucumbers. I add a leaf per jar before I finally close it for storing so that cucumbers keep firm, crispy and crunchy.

People still remember times when they used roasted acorns for food. I will definitely try out one of the old recipes. I am sure that there is enormous power in the seeds of such a powerful tree.

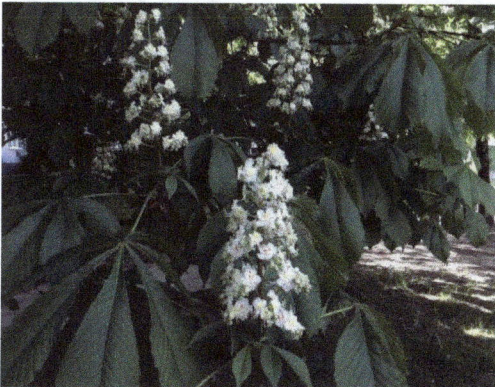

Horse Chestnut

Chestnut
I use the seeds of Horse chestnut. It is my home medicine, my laundry liquid, my dishwasher and material for creative activities with children and grandchildren.

As a home medicine, I make a tincture from fresh chestnut seeds. I fill 1/3 of a jar with chopped chestnut seeds, add high percentage alcohol, keep it tightly closed for at least two weeks, and shake it daily. Then I strain the liquid and pour it into a dark bottle for storing. I use it as a prevention for varicose veins. My father and mother suffered a lot from varicose veins. So far I am very lucky and I have no problems at all. Is it thanks to this tincture or to my habit to sit with legs up, whenever I have a chance....

I love nature and I am really conscious of the damage we humans cause by polluting nature and ourselves, thus I systematically try to replace all the synthetic and nature polluting laundry, washing and cleaning liquids and powders in my home. I want to contribute to preserving nature. I want my grandchildren to learn how to cherish nature, to be able to enjoy the green, the fresh, the beautiful. Telling is one, teaching by example is something else. I try to teach by example.

For my laundry I use either dark green ivy (hedera) leaves, or fresh or dried Sweet William herb or horse chestnut seeds. I cannot imagine laundry with any synthetic powder or liquid anymore. As this is a chapter about chestnut - here is my recipe:

Collect chestnuts, chop them fresh (do not remove the brown shell), dry well and store in tightly closed jars.

For a laundry you pour 300 ml of boiling water onto 3 spoons full of dried chestnuts, let it soak for about 30 minutes, strain the liquid through a sieve and pour it into the washing machine. Do not throw away the thick mass. You can use it once or twice again for washing if you do more laundry in the coming days.

The southern part of Tirol is proud of sweet chestnut (Castanea sativa). They have beautiful, delicious seeds which one can use in so many ways. Every autumn there is a kind of a gourmet festival called Törggelen: you drink wine and eat roasted sweet chestnuts together with other specialties of the region like ham and cheese and bacon....Many people come just for that. It is very popular. And roasted chestnuts are so delicious.

Walnut
Walnut is valued not only for the delicious nuts. I collect the leaves, the green shell of the nuts and the nuts, of course.

The leaves and green outer layer of the nuts have a lot of tannins which make them valuable as home medicine. I add them to my mixtures for stomach problems, spasms or light diarrhea.
My favorite is the nut! I add them to my apple pie (apple strudel), or baked apples. Or have nuts as a snack while hiking. Have you tried to store nuts in honey? It's delicious.

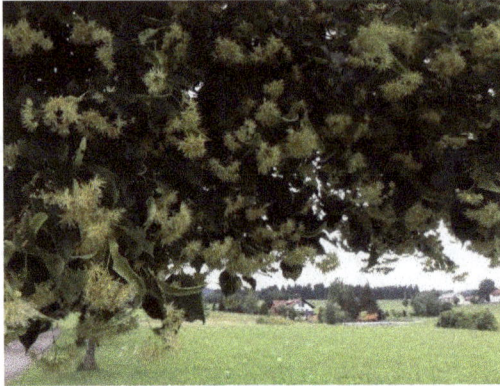

Lime

Lime
Father Künzle did not mention Lime tree in his book, but I definitely want to say many good words about this precious tree. This was the first wild leaf I ate in my life. We had a very good nursery teacher and she showed us young lime leaves in spring. I think I was three years old and I still remember when we tried the leaves for the first time and how soft, mild and delicious they were. It makes me think of the importance of introducing plants to very young children. The smaller the better. And not only the edible plants, but also the dangerous, the poisonous ones, so that the child knows and distinguishes them. When I run my Workshops, I always encourage mothers to bring their children. Well, they are really interested in the plant world. Sometimes even more than their mothers.

And the scent of lime blossoms! It is definitely the best scent in the world for me When I was younger, when I still believed in buying perfumes, I was looking for this scent. No, they said, it is not possible to conserve the natural scent of a lime blossom.

I am looking for blossoming lime trees every early summer and then I do not only collect the flowers, but inhale, inhale this wonderful scent.

The lime blossoms are in all my mixtures for cold, flu. If one is ill, one sweats a lot after drinking lime blossom tea. If one is healthy, one would not sweat.

The leaves have mucus which soothes the pain in the sore throat. I simply chew a leave and let mucus cover my throat.

Limes used to be very important to Germanic peoples. It would grow in the village squares. It was a place for important meetings, village courts, gathering of young people and first kisses.

Hawthorn
I would also like to say a few words about Hawthorn. It is such a useful tree for the elderly. By now it is a very well researched plant, and it is widely used for heart problems and circulation. I always collect blossoms, leaves and fruit and store them dried. As I have no heart and circulation problems, I sometimes add them to my herbal mixtures, especially in wintertime, but I do that as a prevention, a precaution, as additional help to my heart. It is also good for bringing down the high blood pressure. But if anyone has heart or circulation problems - one should ask for a doctor's advice. As Father Künzle suggests, first look for the reason. Why is your heart not as strong as it should be, then think of what you can do. Hawthorn might be one of the solutions.

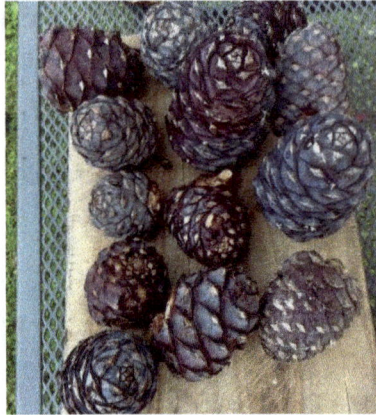

Stone Pine Cones

Alpine pine and other conifers.
Father Künzle mentioned conifers more than once in his book.
They are the source of health. "Forest bathing" is a new, modern
way of restoring or maintaining health. Father Künzle did not
use this term, but what he suggested was very similar to a
modern "forest bathing": in case of a nervous breakdown look
for calmness in a pine forest, for weakness or even tuberculosis,
go out and breath as deep as you can, or fill the room with
conifer twigs. And the higher in the Alps the trees grow, the
better they are. Thus the dwarf mountain pine, creeping high up,
or Austrian/Swiss stone pine growing only beyond 1800 m are
the best ones.

Here in the Austrian and Swiss Alps stone pine is highly
cherished for many reasons. The wood is very hard, that is why
living rooms "Stube" used to be made of stone pine: paneling,
ceilings, furniture. Recently scientists proved that stone pine
wood slows down the heartbeat and, in this way, extends life.
Since this was published, there has been a boom of stone pine
bedrooms. The prices of the wood went up.... and local people
have known that for ages. Our neighbor, a carpenter, a person

who loves and cherishes nature and everything that is natural has built his whole house from stone pine wood.

The stone pine is a special plant: stone pine wood is used for furniture or paneling, stone pine nuts are an excellent food; stone pine oil - a wonderful medicine, stone pine wood shavings in a sleeping pillow calm you down and contribute to a quieter sleep...

Well, I neither have a house or a bedroom of stone pine, but every autumn I collect stone pinecones and make a tincture. It is a nice drink during cold winter evenings, or when you return home from a cold winter walk. I have it for pleasure. It is my favorite tincture.

This is how I make it: the cones for tincture shouldn't be ripe. They have a bluish, violet color. One does not need many: two larger or three smaller cones are enough per one liter of Schnapps or Vodka. I cut cones into slices, put them into a bottle, pour high-quality 40% alcohol, close the bottle, keep it at room temperature for 4-6 weeks, shake the bottle now and then. I do enjoy watching the color turning from light purple into intense red and into dark burgundy. Then I strain the liquid through a thicker cloth and store it for suitable moments to enjoy. Some women add a little bit of sugar and turn it into a sweet liquor to be enjoyed with female friends. Not me. I like pure pinecone tincture.

In my opinion this is a great digestive and helps to avoid respiratory colds ... and has a very good smell.

If there are no stone pines around, one can try making tincture with cones of any pine which are not ripe. It is worth trying.

Final

Father Künzle showed the trees through the eyes of somebody who has not seen the trees. To my mind, it has a deep meaning. We, those, who still live in the luxurious surroundings of trees, woods, forests, take them so naturally. But there are so many areas on the Earth where the trees are rare either because of the natural climate, or because we, humans, have turned forests into deserts, into monoculture farms, into meadows for cattle...

There is a saying that you appreciate the real value of something - be it a human being, an object, a state of mind, or health, or ... a tree, when you lose it. I hope we will never reach the stage, when we will have already lost the vast variety of plants because of our greed, or our ignorance, or indifference. Well, I am an optimist and I believe that we humans will never reach the stage of no return.

I hope that this book will serve its purpose, namely, to help us to stay healthy and to enjoy the vast variety and richness in nature. I hope that not only us, but also our children and grandchildren and many generations after us will be able to enjoy the shades of majestic trees, the beautiful flowers in their natural surroundings, the scent of herbs, and not forget to thank HIM for this beautiful, unique world.

Jolanta Wittib

I live in Tirol in the Austrian Alps, not too far away from where Father Künzle collected his herbs. I run herbal workshops, organize herbal walks and lectures, write and translate. I love learning and I love sharing. I can speak three languages and can read in two more. This enables me to increase my herbal knowledge from different cultures and to pass it on to locals, guests and readers of my blogs and in books.

I studied philology, languages, education management, therefore, for a long time my professional activity focused on teaching, managing, working in educational policy. At that time Herbs and gardening had been my hobby.

At the age of 50, I was ready and able to turn it around. Herbs and gardening became my main occupation. I attended courses on herbs and folk medicine and became a certified herb teacher. Herbs are my food, my medicine, balsam for the soul, nourishment for the spirit. I try out old and new recipes, make my own herbal mixtures, oils and tinctures, introduce new herbs into my life and teach what I myself have learned and tried out.

I joined The Grow Network because I felt that this movement connects people like me: those who grow their own food, medicine, who like sharing and learning not only from each other but also from a large pool of experts.

I am very happy that Judson approached me about this joint project. During the translation I learned a lot from Father Künzle, and by sharing our experiences, I learned a lot from Judson - from his extraordinary knowledge of medicinal plants and ancient herbalists.

If you want to see the herbs described in this book in nature, or just want to chat about herbs, drop me an email:
Jolanta.wittib@gmail.com
Jolanta

Judson Carroll

I am a certified Master Herbalist and Permaculturist from the Blue Ridge Mountains of North Carolina, USA. I began learning about herbs and their uses from the old Appalachian folks, especially the Hicks family of Beech Creek, when I was around 15.

I host the Southern Appalachian Herbal Podcast: Southern Appalachian Herbs (spreaker.com)
I teach free, online herbal medicine classes: Herbal Medicine 101 (rumble.com)
I also write a weekly article on herbs and their properties:
https://southernappalachianherbs.blogspot.com/

My passion is being outside, enjoying the woods, the water and the garden. My mission is to revive the tradition of "folk medicine" in America, so families can care for their own ailments at home, using the herbs God gave us for that purpose. It has been my honor to work with Jolanta on this project.

You can join Jolanta and me on The Grow Network forums – I am a moderator and contributor there. https://thegrownetwork.com/

My email address is southernappalachianherbs@gmail.com

The list of plants

Latin	English	German, Swiss, old Swiss
Abies	Fir tree	Tanne
Achillea millefolium	Yarrow	Schafgarbe
Adiantum capillus-veneris,	the Southern maidenhair fern	Das Frauenhaarfarn
Aegopodium podagraria	Ground elder	Geissfuss
Agropyrum repens	Couch grass	Schliessgras
Alchemilla alpina	Alpine Lady's Mantle	Silbermänteli, Silbermantel
Alchemilla vulgaris	Lady's Mantle	Taumänteli, Frauenmänteli, Mäntelichrut, Muetergottesmänteli, Frauenhilf, Aller Fraue Heil, Sinnau, Frauenmantel
Allium ursinum	Ramsons, Wild garlic	Bärlauch, Rämschelen, Rimschelen
Allium victorialis	Alpine leek	Allermannsharnisch
Alnus glutinosa	Common alder	Erle
Anemonastrum	Buttercup family	Hannenfuß
Anemone coronaria	garden anemone De Caen	Anemone von Caen
Anemone hepatica	Hepatica, American liverwort	Leberblümchen
Anemone ranunculoides	yellow anemone, buttercup anemone	Windröschen
Anthriscus cerefolium	Chervil	Roßkümmi
Angelica archangelica,	garden Angelica	Angelika
Anthyllis vulneraria	Kidney vetch	Echte Wundklee
Aquilegia	Columbine	Akelei
Armoracia rusticana	Horseradish	Meerrettich
Arnica Montana	Arnica	Arnika

Artemisia absinthium	Wormwood	Wermut, Wormet
Arum	Arum	Aron
Aspidium filix	male fern	Farn, Falegata, Filice, Federfarn, Strausfarn, Fötzeln
Asplenium scolopendrium	Hart's tongue fern	Die Hirschzunge
Asplenium trichomanes	Wall fern	Mauerfarn
Atriplex hortensis	Garten orache	Graue Melde
Betula alba, Betula pendula	Birch	Billeche, Birke
Bryophyta	Moss	Moos (Moes), Fenstermoos, Kranzmoos
Buxus sempervirens	The common box	Buchs
Calendula officinalis	Pot marigold	Ringelblume
Caltha palustris	Marsh marigold, kingcup	Dotterblume
Calystegia sepium, convolvolus sepium	Bindweed	Wilde winde
Capsella bursa pastoris	shepherd's purse	Hirtentäschli
Capillary veneris	The maidenhair fern	Frauenhaar
Carum carvi	Caraway	Kümmi, Kümmel
Castanea sativa	Sweet chestnut	Kastanienbaum, Edelkastanie
Centaurium erythraea	Common centaury	Tausengüldenkraut
Cerastium, stellaria	Mouse-ear chickweed	Sternmiere
Cetraria islandica	Iceland moss	Cyprian, Renntierflechte
Chelidonium majus	Greater celandine	Schöllkraut
Cichorium intybus	Chicory	Wegwarte
Clematis vitalba	Old man's beard	Niele, Waldrebe

Colchicum	Meadow saffron	Zeitlose
Convulvus	Bindweeds	Winden, Windeln
Corylus avellana	Common Hasel	Haselnuss
Cyclamen	Cyclamen	Zyklamen
Dactylis glomerata	Cat grass	Knäuelgras
Dryas octopetala	Mountain avens	Steinchrüchtere, Silur, Silberwurz
Dryopteris filix	Fern	Farn
Dryopteris filix mas	Wood fern	Wurmfarn
Equisetum arvense	Common Horsetail	Katzenschwanz, Schachtelhalm, Zinnkraut
Eriophorum	Cotton grass	Wollgrass
Euphorbia	Spurge	Wolfsmilch
Euphrasia rostkoviana	Eyebright	Augentrost, Augstenzieger
Fagus sylvatica	common beech	Buch
Ficaria verna	Lesser celandine, pilewort	Wiesenstern
Filipendula ulmaria	Meadowsweet	Geißbart, Spierstaude, Moorgeissbart, Mädesüss, Geißleite, Wiesengeißbart
Foeniculum vulgare	Fennel	Fenchel, Genchel
Fragaria vesca	Wild strawberry	Wilde Erdbeere
Galium odoratum	the sweetscented bedstraw	Waldmeister
Galium verum	Lady's bedstraw	Chrüglichrut, echtes Labkraut
Gentiana lutea	Great yellow Gentian	Gelber Enzian
Geranium robertianum	Herb Robert, cranesbill	Storchschnabel, Storchenschnabel, St Katharinenchrut, Gottesgnadenchrut,

		Gotesgnadenkraut,
Geum reptans/ urbanum	Creeping avens	St Benediktskraut, Nagelchrut, Nägelichrut, Benediktenkraut, Aller Welt Heil,
Glechoma hederacea	Ground ivy	Gundelrebe, Gundermann
Globularia cordifolia	the heart-leaved globe daisy	Weihwedel
Globularia major und minor	The large and the small Globularia	Weihwedel
Glycyrrhiza glabra	Liquorice	Echtes Süßholz
Gnaphalium	Cudweeds	Katzentöpli
Hieracium alpinum	Alpine hawkweed	Alpen-Habichtskraut
Hieracium murorum	wall hawkweed	Wald-Habichtskraut
Hypericum perforatum	St John's Wort	Johanniskraut
Ilex aquifolium	holly, common holly, English holly	Stechpalme
Imperatoria ostruthium	Masterwort	Horstrinze, Meisterwurz
Juglans regia	English walnut	Nußbaum, Walnuss
Juniperus communis	Juniper	Wacholder, Reckolder
Lamium album	White deadnettle	Weiße Taubnessel
Lamium galeobdolon	Yellow archangel	Goldnessel
Lamium purpureum	Red dead- nettle	Purpurrote Taubnessel
Leontopodium nivale	Edelweiss	Edelweiss
Lycopodium	Stagshorn moss	Bärlapp, Kirchenmoos, Läuskraut
Malva sylvestris	Common mallow	Chäslichrut, Malve
Matricaria chamomilla	Scented mayweed, wild or German chamomile	Kamille
Melissa officinalis	Balm, lemon balm	Melisse, Zitronenmelisse

Mentha	Garden mint	Gartenmünze
Mentha aquatica	Water mint	Wassermünze
Mentha arvensis	Wild mint	Ackermünze, Ackerminze
Mentha piperita	Peppermint	Pfefferminze
Meum mutellina	Alpine lovage	Muttern
Milfoil	Yarrow	Schafgarbe
Ononis spinosa	Spiny restharrow	Hauhechel, Wiberhächle, Türkrnbart
Origanum	Oreganum	Dost
Origanum majorana	Marjoram	Marjoran
Origanum vulgare	Wild marjoram	Wilder Marjoran
Parthenocissus inserta	Young thicket kreeper	Jungernreben
Petasites vulgaris, Petasites hybridus, Tussilago, Petasites	Butterbur	Pestwurz, Sandblaggen, Schneggenblaggen, Berghuflattich
Petroselinum crispum	Parsley	Peterli
Peucedanum ostruthium	Masterwort	Meisterwurz, Horstrinze
Picea abies	European spruce	Rottanne
Pinus mugo	Dwarf Mountain pine	Legföhre, Steinforre, Tschuppen
Pimpinella anisum	Anise	Aenis
Pimpinella saxifraga	Burnet saxifrage	Bibernell, Bockswurzel, Bibernelle
Plantago alpina	Alpine plantain	Rißen, Ritz
Plantago lanceolata	Ribwort Plantain	Spitzwegerich, Rossrippli
Plantago major	Broadleaf plantain	Wegeliballe, Ballentätsch
Plantago media	Hoary plantain	Wiesenwägerich,
Polygonum aviculare	Knotgrass	Steinknötterich, Knötterich
Populus	Cottonwood	Pappel

Populus alba	silver poplar	Silberpappel
Potentilla anserina	Silwerweed	Gänsafingerkraut
Potentilla aurea	dwarf yellow cinquefoil	Goldenes Fünffingerkraut
Potentila erecta	Tormentil	Blutwurz
Potentilla reptans	creeping cinquefoil,	Fünffingerkraut
Potentilla tormentilla	Tormentil	Blutwurz
Primula veris/officinalis	Cowslip	Schlüsseli, Schlüsselblume
Pseudevernia furfuracea	Tree moss	Baummoos
Pulmonaria officinalis	Lungwort	Lungenkraut
Quercus robur	Oak tree	Eiche
Ranunculus	Buttercup	Hahnenfuß
Ranunculus aquatilis	common water-crowfoot	Magdalena Blume, Wasserhahnenfuß
Ranunculus repens	creeping buttercup	Kriechende Hahnenfuß
Rosa canina	Dog rose	Hundrose, Hagebutte
Rosmarinus officinalis	Rosemary	Rosmarin
Rubus fruticosus	Blackberry	Brombeere
Rubus idaeus	Raspberry	Himbeeren
Ruta murorum, Asplenium ruta-muraria	Wall fern	Mauerraute
genus Salix	Willow, sallow, osier	Weide
Salix alba	White willow	Weide Willows, also called sallows and osiers, form the genus Salix
Salvia officinalis	Sage	Salbei
Sambucus nigra	Elder	Holunder

Sambucus ebulus	Danewort	Attich, wilder Holder
Sanguisorba officinalis	Great burnet	Blutstillerin
Sanicula europaea	Sanicle	Sanikel
Sempervivum	Housleek	Hauswurz
Senecio cordatus	alpine ragwort	Alpen-Greiskraut
Senecio fuchsii	wood ragwort	Fuchs-Kreuzkraut, heidnisch Wundkraut,
Senecio vulgaris	Common groundsel	Ackerdistel
Solidago virga aurea	Goldenrod	Goldrute
Sorbus aucuparia	Rowan, mountain ash	Vogelbeere
Spiraea ulmaria	Meadowsweet	Geißbart, Geißleite, wilder Hirsch,
Stellaria Media	Chickweed	Vogelmiere, Vögelichrut, Hahnerdarm, Sternblüemli, Vogelkraut
Stuckenia pectinata	sago pondweed or fennel pondweed	Kamm-Laichkraut, Böner
Symphytum officinale	Common comfrey	Beinwell, Wallwurz
Taraxacum officinale	Dandelion	Löwenzahn, Schwiblume
Thymus serpylum	Breckland thyme, wild thyme	Thymian, Feldthymian
Tormentilla	Tormentil	Tormentill
Triticum repens, Elymus repens	Couch Grass	Schließgras
Tussilago farfara	Coltsfoot	Huflattich, Hutblaggen, Märzblüemli,
Urtica dioica	Common nettle	Brennnessel
Vaccinium myrtillus	Bilberry, European blueberry	Heidelbeeren
Valeriana officinalis	Common Valerian	Baldrian
Verbascum	Mullein	Königskerze

Veronica fruticulosa	speedwell	Halbstrauch Ehrenpreis
Veronica officinalis	Health Speedwell	Ehrenpreis
Viola odorata	Sweet violet	Veilchen, Beieli
Viscum album	Mistletoe	Mistel
Zea	Corn silk, corn beard	Maisbart

www.ingramcontent.com/pod-product-compliance
Lightning Source LLC
Chambersburg PA
CBHW050651270326
41927CB00012B/2971